Praise for *Yoga and the Twelve-Step Path*

"You don't need to be a 'yogi' for your recovery to benefit from this wonderful book. Kyczy Hawk shares practical strategies gleaned from years of yoga study and recovery. You will want to read, study, and practice these techniques and then share them with others in recovery. This book will deepen your recovery and sense of serenity, as it has mine."

Rosemary Tisch, Director, Prevention Partnership International
Lead Author, *Celebrating Families!*

"Yoga and the Twelve-Step Path *is both an invitation and a profound gift. For anyone struggling with addiction, this book could be life-saving and certainly soul-saving. Conscious and cautionary, Ms. Hawk speaks to us as an authentic and powerful teacher who offers up her own compelling story in service to others. With quiet grace, clear direction, and the wisdom of experience, she gently guides the reader along a logical path to health, wellness, and spiritual awakening."*

Mary Lynn Fitton, Founder, The Art of Yoga Project

"Kyczy Hawk has made an important contribution to the field of yoga and addiction recovery. The work and practices laid out in Yoga and the Twelve-Step Path *offer supports to anyone suffering from addiction or anyone who knows someone who is. This book is highly recommended on the journey to recovery."*

Rolf Gates, Teacher and Author, *Meditations from the Mat: Daily Reflections on the Path of Yoga*

"Kyczy Hawk speaks compassionately from her own experience with addiction as she explores the parallels between yoga and the twelve-step path, weaving together a practical guide for enhanced healing. This is a wonderful, life affirming resource! This book offers a comprehensive understanding of yogic concepts, practices, and philosophy, including the eight limbs of raja yoga, which endorse the ideals presented in recovery meetings, and Ayurveda medicine as it relates to addiction. Thank you, Kyzcy, for creating a bridge for those in recovery to discover yoga and those in yoga to understand addiction."

Annalisa Cunningham, Author, *Healing Addiction with Yoga*

"Coming from the depths of her own experience of addiction, and her practice and study of yoga, Kyczy has written an eminently practical book showing how the application of an integrated yoga practice complements, enhances, and enables recovery through the twelve-step approach. In a culture where addiction is endemic, this warm and heartfelt work will be helpful for those battling addiction, as well as students and teachers of yoga."

Bidyut K. Bose, PhD, Executive Director, Niroga Institute

Yoga and the Twelve-Step Path

KYCZY HAWK

YOGA

— AND THE —

Twelve-Step Path

CENTRAL RECOVERY PRESS

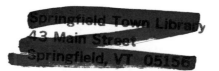

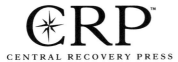

CENTRAL RECOVERY PRESS

CENTRAL RECOVERY PRESS

Central Recovery Press (CRP) is committed to publishing exceptional materials addressing addiction treatment, recovery, and behavioral healthcare topics, including original and quality books, audio/visual communications, and web-based new media. Through a diverse selection of titles, we seek to contribute a broad range of unique resources for professionals, recovering individuals and their families, and the general public.

For more information, visit www.centralrecoverypress.com.

Central Recovery Press, Las Vegas, NV 89129

Publisher: Central Recovery Press
             3321 N. Buffalo Drive
             Las Vegas, NV 89129

18 17 16 15 14 13 12   1 2 3 4 5

ISBN-13: 978-1-936290-80-2 (trade paper)
ISBN-10: 1-936290-80-4

ISBN-13: 978-1-936290-88-8 (e-book)
ISBN-10: 1-936290-88-X

Cover design, interior design and layout by Sara Streifel, Think Creative Design
Author photo by Susan Stojanovich
Yoga illustrations/photos by Della Calfee

TO MY SEMINAL TEACHERS
SHASTA AND SHANNON.

TO MY FRIEND AND HUSBAND BILL.

NAMASTE.

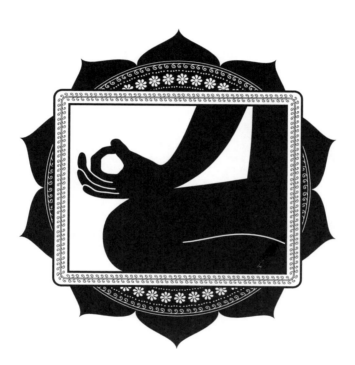

Table of Contents

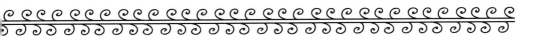

Acknowledgments

There is a Sanskrit word, *guru*, which means "teacher," or, in a more specific sense, someone who takes you from dark to light. There have been many people in my life who have taken me from dark to light personally, in one facet of my life or in many. There are people, too, who have taken this project from dark to light, and I would like to thank them here.

❋   ❋   ❋

My recovery meetings provide me with the quiet voices of struggle and success, and I love my home group, the "In the Solution Group," here in San Jose, California. I am grateful to my sponsors, Mary H. (deceased) for having helped me bring my family back into my life, and Bonnie R. for her support and teaching me about compassion. My adjunct guide, Susan Montana, has been with me the whole time, giving me encouragement and challenging my assumptions about life. Thank you. My sponsees teach me more about myself and the pain of becoming real than any other source. Thank you.

I have a group of yoga teachers who have contributed to both the questions and the answers in my yoga practice and to the information contained in this book. Some laid the groundwork, some enhanced the quest, and others provided resources and structure for this material. Sarla Walter and Kate Walsh gave me my foundation in the yoga practice and principles. Annalisa Cunningham started me on my journey in putting the road of recovery and the path of yoga together. Durga Leela, a teacher and true guru, gave me so much information about taking the tools of *ayurveda* in concert with yoga and recovery to create a self-soothing plan of personal care and enlightenment. Nikki Myer is amazing and generous. She has never held back in offering her help, her wisdom, and the tools she has developed for reaching those who suffer from addiction. Kent Bond has enhanced my physical practice immeasurably, and the quiet weekly talks have helped me discover how the principles of yoga and my recovery program can really be applied to all facets of life. Bonnie Maeda has been my guru and my friend for many decades. She has walked down a complicated and challenging road in life and has shared the process with an open heart. She was the first to expose me to lessons from the mat including the importance of a private practice and the benefits of meditation. She did this all by example. I love you and thank you all.

❋   ❋   ❋

To my students, from those whom I have met only once to those who have met with me for the last several years, I have learned so much from you. Together we have explored the physical, emotional, and spiritual quest of total recovery one day at a time, on one mat at a time. In the cafeterias, meeting halls, basements, and studios you have taught me with your enthusiasm that the benefits of a yoga and breath practice are real, that each step lives in each pose, and that all the principles of yoga do live in a recovery program. Thank you for showing up and showing me the way.

Kids, Bill, Mike and Meridith, and all my cousins—I have a family now. Thanks to my Aunt Audie, who gave me unconditional love and support. She also gave me a wonderful sign I keep on my bookcase: "Thank You for Being." What more could one ask? Over the past years I have been able to mend my relationships and develop healthy interactions with you all. You have given me support in practicing self-forgiveness, self-love, and self-care in my road to recovery. This support then extended through the last several years as I paced around, studied, wrote, took classes and workshops, wrote again, doubted, and finally committed to this book. Life is an amazing journey and you have been my travel mates. Thank you.

❋   ❋   ❋

Finally, thanks to the "midwives" who have taken this from dog-eared notes and typed ramblings to a real book: John Nelson, my first advocate and editor out there in Hawaii. We worked via this wonderful tool—the Internet—to help my book grow up. It worked!!! Thank you. Devra Jacobs, my energetic agent, who was able to match me and my work with a great publishing house in double-quick time. How is that even possible? Thank you. Della Calfee, who was creative and patient in taking all the photos found in the pose guide. She made that task both possible and fun. Susan Stojanovich got me to sit still long enough to have some head shots taken. What a fun time that turned out to be. Thank you. Helen O'Reilly and the folks at Central Recovery Press who have been supportive and kind to this new author who did not know the ropes. What gentle guides. Thank you.

❋   ❋   ❋

I am more grateful than I can express for the journey of getting to this moment. The rest, as they say, is gravy.

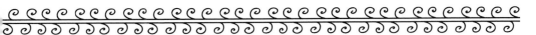

Introduction

Twelve-step programs offer addicts an effective and supportive road map to recovery from addiction in any of its manifestations. The twelve-step process of recovery addresses spiritual and emotional healing, and, as outlined in recovery literature, is used in rehabilitation facilities, between counselors/sponsors and clients/sponsees, and in recovery meetings worldwide. However, aside from acknowledging that medical help should be sought for physical problems, and the recognition that abstinence usually leads to improved health, there is not much in the way of guidance for specific physical rehabilitation in the recovery literature.

Outside of sustained abstinence or mindfulness modification, none of the Twelve Steps is presented to address the physical impact and need for physical healing from the disease of addiction. Yoga is far more than a physical activity; it moves one mindfully into the body, breath, and consciousness of movement. This physical awareness can lead to greater understanding of the emotions and the mind. In my experience, the self-awareness that is needed for full recovery starts with physical attunement; what we find out about ourselves "on the mat" can lead to self-discovery off the mat. I wrote this book to help address the lack of specific direction for physical well-being that I perceived in the program of twelve-step recovery.

Experts agree that abstinence alone is not sufficient to result in long-term recovery. Mental, spiritual, and physical healing have to take place as well. Ceasing the activities of smoking, drinking, and legal or illegal drug use, as well as such behaviors as gambling, abusive Internet gaming, watching online porn, or other manifestations of addiction, is but one step to recovery and health. While the Twelve Steps lead through emotional healing and into the spiritual realm, yoga starts with the physical and takes you through the mental and emotional to the spiritual, and together they unify you—body, mind, and spirit.

I am aware that neither yoga nor the rooms of recovery can address the extremes of physical recovery. The health condition (both mental and physical) of the individual when he or she enters recovery will determine if traditional medical and/or psychological interventions are required. Some people suffering from addiction may have other co-occurring disorders or psychological problems. If extreme, these need to be addressed by medical professionals. These people may enter the rooms of recovery through the advice of their doctors. Other people have walked into a recovery meeting from off the street, where no official intervention—legal, medical, or other encouragement—was needed, outside of a life going to hell fast.

The program of recovery upon which all "anonymous" twelve-step groups are based brings together a community of people who have decided to join one another on the path of wellness. They follow the philosophy of the Twelve Steps and have incorporated most, if not all, of the program suggestions from the recovery literature on a consistent basis. The program guidelines suggest maintaining involvement in the recovery group, as well as working on an individual basis with a more seasoned person, a sponsor. The Twelve Steps help one to become more self-aware and to refresh or acquire and incorporate certain ethics of behavior. There is an invitation to connect or reconnect with a Higher Power, to develop or rekindle a spiritual life. The development of a relationship with a Higher Power may result in closer ties with an organized religion, or in developing a richer intimate relationship, or it may lead to a private connection with a deeper, more abiding spiritual life. The actions and feelings of a person in recovery become more thoughtful and mature, less provocative and fault-finding. The mental capacities expand and improve while the emotional responses and reactions become more measured, restrained, and moral. These are some of the results of working with the Twelve Steps, and they are the underpinnings of health and wellness in a recovering addict.

While one's spiritual and emotional life is improving, the feeling of having reached a "recovery plateau" may occur at some point in one's recovery. There may come a point where negative self-talk doesn't abate, where one's connection with the recovery group feels more tenuous, where the connection to one's Higher Power dims. In addition, one might be experiencing some physical maladies that may require professional help to overcome. The damage that addictive behavior has caused the body—either directly from a substance or indirectly as a result of the activity (nutritional deficits, poor sleep patterns, abnormal weight gain or loss)—needs to be addressed and remedied. While most physical activity is helpful when performed wisely, moderately, and regularly, caution must be taken, as exercise, too, can become an obsession. Exercise, as a purely physical enterprise, can be just that—another source of addiction, even to the detriment of the body. Most exercise is based upon physical prowess: a faster mile, greater weight lifted, increased endurance, or even dedicated concentration on developing the body beautiful. This can become more activity that promotes disconnection from developing mental and spiritual growth and well-being.

Yoga is not just a physical practice. It is a spiritual path with a code of ethics leading to contentment and bliss, and it can lead to spiritual union with one's Higher Power. Excess in the physical practice is seldom encountered, particularly when other yogic practices are combined with the *asanas*, or poses. Each student is guided to practice within his or her capacity, to move into poses that challenge but do not harm the body. In fact, moderation can be part of the lessons that are taught on the mat. There are classes with more of a physical focus, some more extreme or challenging yogas, that can be taken; these often do not include a spiritual component. If there is a spiritual longing in an individual, exclusively physical practices may not provide lasting satisfaction. Yoga that includes all facets of the philosophy will be more fulfilling in the long run and more effective for those in recovery. I was drawn to these classes, which made a yoga class more like a meeting, where I felt comfortable and accepted just the way I was, with the invitation to become more like my best self. It was an opportunity for me, with guidance, to quiet the negative self-talk and again practice the principles that made me whole. The breath practices helped to calm my mind and soothe my body. In time, tools like stretching, breathing, and mind/body awareness became part of my daily stock in trade, allowing me to be more myself in my daily activities when faced with challenges, and to improve my relationships.

While a dedicated yoga study which includes all the facets of the philosophy enhances recovery from addiction, not everyone has a desire to become a *Vedic* scholar. My experience with the practice of yoga began as a physical pursuit. With the aid of true yogis (persons who practice yoga), my understanding very rapidly moved from the physical to include the emotional and spiritual. The yoga philosophy was taking me deeper into my recovery steps, and that journey was beginning to relieve my suffering. The more similarities I found between these lineages, the more I felt supported and able to expand my recovery. However, I was unable to find yoga teachers who could help me draw these parallels. At the beginning of my journey, there was only one published author who also held retreats on the subject. I immediately made contact and studied with her, and yet still I craved more. I needed a road map. I found more practitioners in the next few years who were also struggling to combine the practice of yoga, its philosophy, and the program of recovery. I have learned from them all and have come up with a teaching style that is my own. I also have a desire to share this journey with others, to help draw the connections between these two worlds—the ancient and the new—so that they, too, may investigate the path and benefit from the resources. This is meant to lay the groundwork for a lifetime of curiosity and exploration. The paths are not parallel; they are interwoven. Sponsors may not be well versed in yoga, and yoga teachers may not understand the fatal illness that is addiction. It is the addict him- or herself who must bridge the two disciplines or philosophies.

I have written this book to introduce readers to yoga's ideas and concepts, draw the parallels to the recovery path, and invite readers to practice this awareness on their yoga mat and in their lives. I also include some basic postures to start with, but the reader is encouraged to find a yoga class and teacher in order to expand this practice. Like recovery itself, yoga is versatile and meets you where you are; it also incorporates the key idea of sponsorship—that of learning from the more experienced person, someone who has been down the path before you. The practice of yoga has something to offer to the newly sober as well as those further down the road of recovery.

Addiction is a disease that has mental, physical, and spiritual components. Robert Birnberg calls alcoholism/addiction "perhaps, the first truly holistic disease."[1] As such, addiction requires a threefold remedy: a physical, mental, and spiritual wellness plan. While addiction cannot be cured, the deleterious effects can be halted. The multifaceted practice of yoga mirrors the suggestions of a twelve-step program: this book includes details and practical application of this tradition for the person in recovery.

When I first started practicing yoga, I was stiff, my joints were congested, I ached in the poses, and my breath was short and labored. I asked myself why I was enduring this challenge. My teacher continued to advise me not to overreach—to do my best but to work within comfort, to find my breath and work there. One day, as I was in a forward fold, something released. The teacher was talking about the strength reserves we each had and how we could find them in our practice when we listened. I burst into tears as something in my hips let go, and I realized I could be strong without being isolated; I could stand on my own two feet while being taught, and I did not need to go it alone. What a new concept! I have no idea where the thoughts or the tears came from. All I know is that there was tightness and resistance one moment, and softness and acceptance the next. Yoga practice forged the path for this moment of integration.

Those suffering with addiction often yearn for a proper way to release pent-up energies, fill a psychic hole, or relieve emotional pain trapped inside them. These psychic injuries can be traced to emotional, physical, and spiritual past harms. Yoga is an ideal modality to address the physical recovery. Yoga *asana,* or pose, practice has many forms and styles: there is a yoga tradition and exertion level that will appeal to almost every person. People in recovery need to release toxins that have been stored in their bodies over the years. They need to release pain and trauma trapped in their muscles and joints. Uncomfortable physical sensations—tightness in the shoulders, neck, back, hips, and legs—reflect stress that has been stored in habitual ways and areas. These negative feelings are often actually lodged in their bodies, muscles, and joints. Yoga offers many specialized practices that identify these areas and provide a process for their release. "Joint and gland" exercises, TRE (trauma release exercises), muscle work, and other integral yoga practices focus on certain areas known to store trauma and release the "issues in our tissues," as Nikki Meyer, founder of Y12SR, has called them.

Reiki therapy, the Alexander Technique, and the science of somatics all address the concept that past traumas and injuries live in real time in our muscles, tendons, and ligaments. These past traumas influence how we carry ourselves and use our bodies. There is a need to release these energetic obstructions in order to be free of the impact of these past events, which affect how we think and feel now. The stress and the pain can build and prevent one from experiencing the full benefits of recovery. While deep muscle and tension releases can be found after a period of yoga practice, stress relief in the body and mind can be obtained from the first minutes on the mat. Breath work, stretching, and guided relaxation in *sivasana* (final relaxation pose) can bring an immediate sense of inner peace and calm. The science and practice of yoga therapy is used to address a wide variety of illnesses and diseases ranging from cancer to athletic injury, multiple sclerosis to depression. While specialized yoga techniques are useful, all progressive *hatha* yoga classes can lead the person and the body into balanced health. Given that depression, anxiety, and insomnia can be greatly ameliorated through the physical practice of yoga, addiction recovery and yoga are a natural fit.

At the same time I was starting to practice yoga in studios, I also practiced at home. This home practice wasn't satisfying over the long haul, as I was getting used to the pose shapes without the benefit of personal instruction and without the company of a yoga community. Developing a personal practice is important, but not when it supports isolation rather than community. Loneliness is a hallmark of the disease of addiction, a sign of potential relapse, and a condition of which I needed to be wary. Finding a community with the benefits of a teacher who provides both wisdom and guidance, in addition to other like-minded students with stories to share, is what I needed. This is also beneficial when feelings or responses to the physical releases need comforting and company. This book does not give you the total practice of yoga—there are other detailed texts for that. In fact, my suggestion would be to work with a skilled instructor who can teach the yoga poses in mindful concert with the benefits of recovery. This book does give you a plan, a way of looking at your life so that you can bring these exquisite tools into your kit of spiritual tools, expanding your resources to alleviate pain and prevent relapse. Ultimately, the journey is exclusively that of the student, but wise company can remove some of the pain of isolation.

Along with the health benefits from the physical exercise, there are the other aspects of yoga that can contribute to recovery and ongoing well-being. When I first got into recovery, I was at a loss for ways to take care of myself. I did not realize what a toll my irregular hours, uneven eating habits, poor sleep, and poor healthcare had taken on my body. I heard in the recovery rooms that one should not become too "hungry, angry, lonely, or tired," or HALT, as we refer to it. It makes good practical sense, but I was unskilled at noticing the signs of distress. I overate or forgot to eat; I was plagued with insomnia and indigestion. I had children, and while I understood healthy cooking and nutrition for them, I was unable to apply these principles to myself. When I first came into recovery, I was unable to walk the distance of a city block and was bankrupt in all areas of my life. I did not understand self-care at all. Addiction provided a distraction from daily life, until it had become my daily life. It had become a substitute for all manner of genuine human interaction and a replacement for authentic feelings. Over the course of time, healthy ways of addressing life's issues and desires were lost. Recovering from addiction can leave a tremendous hole in one's abilities to respond to the vicissitudes of life.

Yoga can offer tools to address feelings, thoughts, and actions. These yogic solutions are very similar to those found in recovery programs. They expand upon existing models of recovery that involve intellectual, emotional, and spiritual self-exploration. Yoga provides additional tools that are congruent with the principles of the twelve-step philosophy and include body and breath awareness. Becoming aware of body tones or feelings can lead to greater awareness of the physical conditions that lead to stress, tension, and possibly eventual relapse. Trauma and pain memories stored in the body can ignite unconscious thought patterns and reactions. These feelings can influence perceived choices and impair decision making. The somatic training of yoga postures and the skills of quieting the mind can lead one into a more refined perception of these negative states of being. Becoming aware of how the body feels in the postures can expand to a greater knowledge of how the body and mind are feeling off the mat, when out in life. Not only can yoga release the impact of stored memories, but a regular practice can enhance positive neurological patterns that can sustain us in health.

One must learn to eat when hungry—good food in a wise manner. Be aware of approaching anger, and calm your body (posture and breathing) to calm your mind. Discover the issues and find the patience and wisdom to deal with them effectively. Do not isolate—find peers in all areas of your life who are healthful and wise. When you are tired, sleep. Each of these conditions had an answer in addictive behavior. Finding the answer in a healthful manner for mind, spirit, and body can be achieved when practicing yoga.

Developing a reverential attitude toward self and a sense of being able to establish boundaries is important. Listening to music that inspires rather than agitates, being aware of the impacts of colors and smells, finding rest rather than stimulation when one is tired—these are all skills that must be practiced in order to be useful and at the ready when needed. Yoga teaches and reinforces the importance of each. Addicts practice total disregard of self for years before gaining recovery. A codependent person will ignore symptoms of illness and disease while carefully attending to the needs of others. People with food addictions will not know the symptoms of hunger or indigestion as they focus on other cues (such as lightness of being for anorexics or the habits of eating and purging for bulimics, for example). They have not learned yet to listen to the senses built into a healthy body. Yoga can begin to make one more aware of these learned shortcomings, and can offer a new way of approaching hunger and eating, caring for others, or filling an unconscious internal void.

Stress is also a major source of relapse. The tools of the twelve-step recovery program, along with the physicality of a regular yoga practice included in *hatha* classes, can prevent stress from accumulating and release stress once it builds. To quote Dr. Steven Melemis, PhD, MD, an authority on addiction and relapse prevention, "There are only a few reasons why people use drugs and alcohol. They use to escape, relax, and reward themselves. In other words, people use drugs and alcohol to relieve tension." Later he states, "Your mind and body relax as a unit because they are in constant communication. Since it's hard to relax your mind, relax your body first, and your mind will follow."[2] This reinforces the definition of addiction outlined in "The Doctor's Opinion" chapter in *Alcoholics Anonymous*, which describes alcoholism as "a manifestation of an allergy" and says that "alcoholism is an illness which only a spiritual experience will conquer."

Developing strategies to deal with negative feelings as they arise is critical to long-term recovery. Yoga teaches us self-awareness and provides the practical tools to identify and relieve tension caused by stress—to relax. The practice of yoga itself can become a reward.

Initially, the goal of recovery is to cease the destructive habit or behavior. As we continue our journey to wellness, we utilize the tools of recovery to identify actions and attitudes that are no longer serving us. The same is true in the practice of yoga, where first we learn the poses, then we learn our bodies. The feelings stored in the body will lead us to a deeper understanding of our reactions and remembrances. Your body lets you in—meaning that you cannot force yourself into right awareness; you move into it. At a certain point your breath will guide you as you become more physically attuned to your own stress level. You are able to sense tension or stress as the result of having experienced relaxation. In recovery programs you learn to note when you are behaving in a dangerous fashion (such as holding on to resentments or developing expectations, identifying when you are feeling fearful or insecure), and then find an appropriate action to take to ameliorate these feelings. This may include calling your sponsor, going to a meeting, or turning to your spiritual guide; so, too, in yoga, you become more mindful at feeling the tensions in the body—the stored anxieties or anger. You can then employ your yoga tools to address them. Moving toward the discomforts and dealing with them are keys to maintaining a recovered life. Avoiding the signs and symptoms of stress and distress can signify the slippery slope into relapse. Having more and healthier choices to employ in these situations can help prevent relapse from happening.

I had searched classes, workshops, retreats, and bookstores in my quest for a process, a method, or an approach to combining *hatha* yoga, yoga philosophy, and the twelve-step recovery path. This combination felt so natural that I was sure others must have already trodden this path and made those discoveries public. While there were a few books and several programs, all of which helped me in my recovery, I felt that they were mostly too esoteric to help others new to the subject. I then took all that I had read and learned and incorporated it into a more basic approach in my yoga classes and workshops. Over the past several years I have brought yoga classes into halfway houses, detention facilities, and church basements as well as yoga studios. Combining the two philosophies with the physical postures and breath work, I have developed a teaching style that brings them all together.

This book will discuss and detail the yogic concepts of the *gunas* (emotional qualities) and the *doshas* (physical and mental qualities). It will explain them in sufficient detail so the reader can use them to begin to evaluate his or her own state of being. This understanding will contribute to helpful identification of the optimum soothing techniques for each unique person. Evaluation questionnaires are included. I have found that knowing myself better, having tools to interpret the patterns of my thoughts and to distinguish what I was feeling, was a key to self-care. Using these tools, I was able to move from the thoughts in my head into the feelings in my heart through compassionate self-love. I was finding a way to both know myself and accept myself the way I am. I was better able to focus on my self-care by using these tools and making these skills and habits more effective and enjoyable, while developing a sustainable system for my personal, unique being.

The twelve-step program leads us into and through the emotional and spiritual damages of addiction to a greater sense of well-being. As one develops an awareness of a Higher Power and gains the trust and faith to depend on it, healing takes on a deeper and more profound nature. With the dislodging of past wrongs and an awareness of personal traits, coping styles, and weaknesses, one can make better choices about future behavior and take actions so as to avoid repeating past errors and wrongs. This journey of emotional and spiritual healing includes development of, or reacquaintance with, certain ethical and moral values. The three basic values taught in the twelve-step programs are honesty, open-mindedness, and willingness. There are other principles such as service and working with others that are also crucial to recovery. These basic standards are expanded upon in the philosophy of yoga.

A study of the various yogas and the limbs of *raja* yoga enhances, endorses, and expands the ideals that are presented in recovery meetings. In *raja* yoga one learns of the restraints (*yamas*), the observances (*niyamas*), breath work, letting go, contemplation, meditation, and union with one's Higher Power in addition to the *hatha* practices. The various classical, well-known yogas—*karma, bhakti, mantra, jnana,* and *raja*—each relate strongly to a piece of the twelve-step recovery programs. *Karma* yoga is the yoga of action and consequences (Steps Four through Seven and Step Ten). *Bhakti* yoga is the yoga of passionate devotion to a Higher Power (Steps Two and Twelve). *Mantra* yoga is a yoga of sound or phrase repetition to achieve union with one's Higher Power (prayers and sayings). *Jnana* yoga is the yoga of reality and study (working all the steps with a sponsor). *Raja* yoga is the path leading to bliss and union with the divine (the steps and traditions augmented with physical recovery). The similarities between aspects of the twelve-step programs and each of the various types of yoga allow for the practice of yoga to support recovery, while deepening and expanding on the systems of belief one learns in the rooms of recovery.

Yoga gives us specific tools to find our true selves. Breath work is critical. It is the foundation of all yogic practices, including the *asana.* Breathing in a deep and sustained manner has beneficial neurological effects. It can change the physical responses to a situation from an instinctual "fight-or-flight" reaction to a more measured and thought-out response. This is a vital change for people who have poor impulse control or the inability to find a mature solution to an immediate problem. Further in meditation, investigating how the mind works, how one's own mind works, is a step in the yoga path. Are you a person who ruminates obsessively on the past? Does your mind travel into the future, anticipating events, or fantasizing about life as it could have been?

Learning what your particular mind does—the ruts of past experiences it travels through, and the habits of future travel it may take—is useful to know. Self-reflection can offer some insight, and this insight can then offer choices on how to act or how to redirect thinking into healthier avenues. Getting bound up in guilt from past actions, or becoming mentally involved in some aspect of a future event that may or may not occur, can be habits that bring about wrong thinking ("stinking thinking," as some in recovery call it). These mental states can lead to relapse. Breath work, practicing the *yama* of nonattachment, taking a physical inventory of the feeling tones in the body, and meditation are all tools that are compatible with programs of recovery, regardless of the manifestation—gambling, relationships, consumerism, or drugs. The mental gymnastics and delusions of addiction are very similar in every addict.

Many inpatient recovery centers offer yoga as part of their treatment plans. There are nonprofit organizations that bring yoga to the incarcerated, the institutionalized, and the disenfranchised. There are programs for at-risk youth and juvenile offenders. The benefits of yoga are being accepted in more and more mainstream locations. This book is for those who want to know a little more about how and why this philosophy is compatible with the goals of health and recovery. It is a guide for people who are in recovery or have left a recovery center and want to continue the practice on their own. Each chapter goes into a yoga practice in detail, drawing on the relationship between yoga and recovery programs. Exercises, breath practices, and *hatha* yoga postures are offered at the end of each section. By practicing these, the reader will gain a working knowledge of the tools and benefits of this ancient and amazing resource: yoga.

INTRODUCTION NOTES

[1] Birnberg, Robert. 2006. *Yoga, Habit, and Freedom from Addiction* [Online]. Available from www.longexhale.com (accessed October 2010).

[2] Melemis, Steven M. *Recovery Skills* [Online]. Available from www. addictionsandrecovery.org (accessed February 2011).

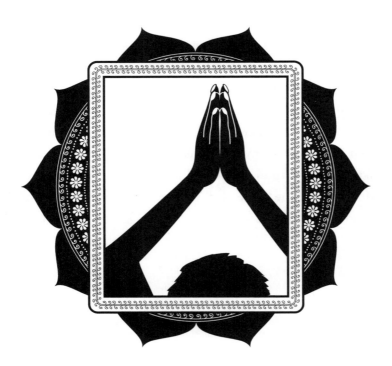

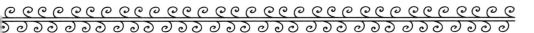

CHAPTER ONE

My Story

SAN FRANCISCO IN THE LATE 1960S. What a place and an era for an alienated, frightened, headstrong teenager. With the heart of a socially conscious rebel and the dependencies of an addict, I was let loose in a city that had the answer to my fears. As early as ninth grade, I got into pot and diet pills; the summer before high school I joined protest marches and drank red wine; high school added acid and other drugs to the mix, and it was off to the races.

Like many, but not all, addicted people, I came from an emotionally impaired home. We moved frequently during my preteen years. My parents were teachers, and we moved from country to country as they obtained contracts with various schools and universities. We children learned to adapt to different countries and languages, never forging close ties due to cultural differences, lack of skills, and the knowledge that we would be leaving in a short while. My mother was an active alcoholic in countries that permitted drinking, and a dry drunk in countries that did not. My father was an angry man who was deeply disenchanted with his career, his family, and his life. My parents were brilliant people, loved by their friends, but unskilled at being parents—part of their tender flaws. That made raising children a challenge for them. They often lived countries apart from each other, and this was the case when I entered my thirteenth year in northern California—the summer that I dove into the world of alcohol and drugs. My mother was searching for recovery herself—a painful journey she did not fully embrace until shortly before I left home. During those years my brother, nine years younger, and my sister, only eighteen months younger, were each as different from me as siblings could be, but I tried to play house and create a "normal" American family without adult supervision. We maintained the house and did the shopping, cooking, and cleaning. My mother tried to reengage as a parent from time to time, but those phases did not last long. When my father returned to the United States, it meant he was unemployed and was depressed and despondent, full of regrets and remorse, which came out as outbursts of anger.

My youthful "controlled drinking and using" meant that I had to be down from my high and semicoherent by late afternoon to cook dinner for the family and do my homework. At that point in my using career, I was still trying to be a good girl. It was a pattern that would follow me through my addiction years. I walked a tightrope between being a good and eager student, friend, and daughter and being a wild, politically active protestor, drinker, and drug user. While I believed strongly in the political protest against the Vietnam War and social change for both racial and gender equality, I was enchanted with drugs, including alcohol. I ended most weekend rallies by going home with some older guy to get high, rather than with a fellow demonstrator or activist to plan for another day's activities.

My bad behavior carried over to my home, where I was an impossible child. On one hand, while managing our household and doing most of the chores, I also tried to parent my younger siblings and mediate the fights between my parents. On the other hand, I was frequently high or drunk, reckless with my health and safety, and truant from school whenever possible. As I said, with my father working out of the country much of the time and my mom suffering with her own demons, I was drawn to the freedom of the streets and the irresponsibility of the urchin life. I ran away from home a couple of times to avoid terrors, real or imagined. I threatened to drop out of high school, but instead I did an accelerated program and graduated early. I was that unsure of my ability to continue the duplicitous life of the good girl/bad girl. I couldn't keep the two lives apart. The compliant student was no longer stronger than the full-blown addict. Soon after graduating from high school at seventeen, I left home.

In and out of junior college, in and out of relationships, taking minimum-wage jobs, and hanging out with the kids who had dropped out of high school, I continued my drug and alcohol use. I did so until I moved to Colorado, but not before getting pregnant. I was sure having a baby would give me structure and purpose. I moved away with the love of my life, hoping that the opportunities near Boulder would keep me straight and allow for us to create a "normal" life. However, "wherever you go—there you are." I was still a depressed, insecure, frightened, dependent girl. I was leaning on him to give me security and focus. I had no real employment skills; I was still a mess. I went back to doing what I knew how to do: the good girl in me did volunteer work at the elementary school, and the addict side worked in the local bar at night.

Pregnancy made me nauseated, and for those months I was unable to drink. I was not a sane person. Being young, with raging hormones, large with child, jealous of all women, and alone in an unknown state, I was unkind and possessive, frightened, and demanding of all. As soon as my daughter was born, I was drinking again. Working in the bar made drinking affordable, and I drank for entertainment, for distraction, and as an excuse for all the hell we put each other through. The relationship with "him" broke up, drama ensued, and another baby was conceived. And "he" was gone.

I returned to school, and this time the pregnancy could tolerate drinking, so I was drunk most of the time. I worked in a bar, tended to my child, went to school, and studied. For five long months, I exhausted my body and mind with this cycle of school, motherhood, and my barmaid job on the weekends. I again came to the edge of insanity, and this time tipped right over. I created a drama to reunite myself and my children with their father (unsuccessfully); I successfully finished my semester at university and moved back to California. I had enlisted the help of friends to bring me back. One woman flew out and drove us back to the Bay Area, while another housed and comforted me until I could find my own place. With public assistance I was able to rent a place with roommates and enroll in college again.

So the good girl wanted to become a good mother and a good student, and to be employable. The bad one found intravenous (IV) drugs. I remained enrolled in school, gave birth to my second child, and had addicts and dealers in the house. I was part of the parent-participation nursery school my daughter attended, was a board member of a local nonprofit, attended single mothers' group meetings, and went to college. I also drank like a fish and used drugs. The three of us—my two children and I—were incredibly fortunate not to have been harmed by others as the result of my lifestyle. Drugs, including alcohol, were now a requirement for daily living. Friends were betrayed and lost forever; my family was disappointed time and time again by broken promises and unreliable agreements. Even doing jobs like house painting for cash seemed beyond my ability. Once again I rushed through school to be certain I could finish—without a job skill but with a diploma.

Relationships with family, friends, and roommates were trashed, and eventually falling in love and moving in with a dealer seemed like a reasonable solution to my using needs.

I was able to keep a receptionist job after college graduation. It was not quite the career I imagined after having earned a BA degree, but I was ill-suited for anything else. I did quit IV drugs, but was now a round-the-clock drinker. My daily cutoff was five a.m.; I had to be at work at eight, and it took three hours for my breath to clear. I worked eight hours a day, picked the children up from preschool, stopped at a small corner market for a quart of rum, and went home to hole up, pretend to be a mom, put the kids to bed, and drink through the night. I did this for several years, breaking down my body, puffing up with the high sugar content of the alcohol, and living on poor food and little sleep. I ended up breaking all promises to my kids about trips to the zoo, the beach, or the park, or even just going outdoors. I even lost track of whether I had fed them at night. I would frequently dress them in dirty clothes, as I often couldn't stop drinking to retrieve the laundry from the laundromat until after it had closed. I became so worn down and paranoid that I could no longer make decisions at a store, make change, or answer the door or phone at home. Work became increasingly challenging, and I was an emotional wreck.

One night I sat on the edge of the bed—no special night or unusual event—when I thought, "I cannot go on, I cannot do this anymore." I was unclear in my mind as to whether "this" referred to taking care of the kids and going to work or to drinking and using. I felt strongly that I could not do both, and if I chose to continue to drink and use, my kids would go, the job would go, and my actual SELF would go— my authentic, genuine, inside soul/self would drift away. I would walk out the door and not return—go into the arms of whoever could or would keep me high. I felt as if I could actually see my core being as a mist floating in front of my eyes; the choice between dissipating or integrating was as fragile as my next breath.

Finally I moved to the phone to call a friend who, as rumor had it, was in recovery. She answered her phone and eagerly agreed to meet me and take me to a meeting the next day. I had my last drink that night, but drugs did not leave me that easily. While I abstained from alcohol for nearly three months, I knew I had to move away from my dealer boyfriend. So I moved to San Jose, hoping that a new town would separate me from my obsessions. My need for him was all balled up with my need for drugs, and I was unable to keep them separate for quite some time. I finally broke up with him, cutting myself off from the supply, and really entered recovery. I had not been honest in my twelve-step meetings about the drug use, so I had not sought support. I slipped one final time, drinking a pint of cough syrup. That was twenty-five years ago. So, though I stepped into the rooms on July 5, 1983, my recovery anniversary is actually April 29, 1985.

During the past two-plus decades I have raised my family, found a career, and seen my parents through their final illnesses and my brother through a life-changing accident. I have made friends with my family and family out of my friends. The road to emotional and spiritual health was not smooth. It was necessary for me to get professional counseling, something I would utilize on occasion for most of my life. I was so shaky in my first recovery meetings that I cannot tell you much about them. Some people can remember with enviable clarity their first meeting, their first work with a sponsor. That was not to be the case for me. I was a mental, physical, emotional, and spiritual wreck.

I had continued to attend meetings almost daily and to work with (and withhold the truth from) my sponsor this whole time. It wasn't until I was ready to establish a "new" recovery date by going out and getting loaded that I realized the danger of keeping my secret. I finally told the truth about my using at a meeting. This I did not do all on my own. My Higher Power had intervened. I heard a woman share who had done the same thing: she had continued to use drugs as she continued to attend twelve-step recovery meetings. I felt nothing but compassion for her; I did not feel pity, and I did not sit in judgment or scorn her. And as I listened and looked around the room, I saw the same emotions on everybody's face: compassion, concern, and care. I stood up with what we call "a burning desire" to share and told everyone my story of self-betrayal. And they loved me, too. Eventually I went to all of my regular meetings, changing my recovery date out loud and feeling humility with that action of amends.

Now I could dig into my steps for a second time with renewed honesty and more self-awareness. While I had made sincere amends the first time through the steps of the program, addressing all the issues and events I could remember at that time, I had a new appreciation for who I had been and who I wanted to be. That gave me a finer comb with which to remove the tangles of my past. It was as if a veil had been lifted between my inner self and others: I could listen with my whole heart and respond honestly from the totality of my being. It also gave me a new place of authenticity to be a sponsor to others. I could "give so freely that which had been given to me"—acceptance and empathy.

With the madness of having lived the "lie of deception" in my early recovery, I truly found the unmanageability of my disease. I realized that I would have to include and rely on a power greater than myself for resolution and guidance, that I could become whole and find my genuine authentic self, and that there were still moral wrong turns to evaluate and evacuate. I needed to know what my spiritual road was and how to proceed. This is an ongoing search, and I am patient. I tried organized religion, I tried me-ism, and I tried "him" again—making my partner my deity. This also does not work, and is an unfair burden on a partner and an unrealistic source of inspiration and approval. In my journey I have discovered that the real source of inspiration and approval comes from inside, and is based on my spiritual life.

We are taught in recovery that we need to find a Higher Power that we are comfortable with and develop a relationship with it. While much of the writing in the basic texts of recovery reads from a traditional monotheistic model, we are given the option to find our own spiritual path in any manner or direction we wish. Twelve-step pioneer Bill Wilson averred that the program "contained spiritual principles that members of any and every religion could accept, including the Eastern religions" (*Pass It On: The Story of Bill Wilson and How the AA Message Reached the World*, p. 283). As a result of this search, I am on a very comfortable path now of worshiping the divinity in all of us. I have my group of wise people who demonstrate the life I want to lead and advise me along the way. I have been able to take the principles from the twelve-step recovery program into my daily practice, and to weave them into my daily activities and my relationships with my husband, children, and grandchildren. I have also been able to work them into my career choices and my relationship with myself.

Once abstinence was firmly a part of my life, once I had dealt with the wreckage of my past, and once I was solidly practicing the principles of the twelve-step program in my daily life, I still had an inner landscape to explore. Moving down the path in recovery, I found the need to heal my body, to get into movement and rehabilitate my stagnant physiology. As my children grew up, I had more opportunities to be on my own and could walk, try gym classes, and even take a dance class. Each of these had physical health as a focus, and I became more fit and strong (initially I could only manage to walk around my block, and eventually I was able to run a ten-mile race). Physical health was only one aspect of the recovery I sought. I went to a church and hung around with people who had a spiritual life and a spiritual quest. I belonged to an antiwar/nonviolence group. I was patching together solutions to my overall needs for a holistic answer to my deeper longings. I was unsure what physical discipline could combine with my need to move into my body, spirit, and recovery. Then I found yoga.

I do not have a flexible body, but I do have a flexible mind. I am aware of my physical limitations, but my desire for the integration of body, mind, and spirit has no such limits. I was afraid of stepping into a yoga studio for fear of not fitting in, of lack of capability, and of being "not as good as." I actually had to try a few yoga studios to find one with a heart, the one that had room for the inquiring, uncertain student in me. I was fortunate enough to have teachers who brought attention to the breath as well as the postures. They taught the principles of working within your own capacity and accepting yourself the way you are, and they taught integration of spirit, body, and mind during final relaxation. These skills are useful on the mat and in your life.

Each class allowed me to release more and more stiffness and tension. My shoulders, which were often drawn up to my ears, began to descend as I released the weight of the world I had been carrying for so long. Once I learned to identify and let go of tension, I was able to replace that with strength—strength and energy to deal with "life on life's terms" rather than fighting, resisting, and controlling.

I had heard and read enough to know that yoga was more than just the postures, and that there was a reason for the breath work and meditative aspect, and that the practice could provide me with a doorway to further integration. Recovery had reached a plateau, and my spiritual seeking had moved me away from a church—but toward something more defined than "Good Orderly Direction" or "Group of Drunks/Druggies" (as some in recovery say). I was definitely looking for a deeper connection. Yoga is not a religion; it is a spiritual practice. My continuing journey had to include a deeper sense of self-knowledge and an embrace of the divine around and within me. This came to me through the smoothness of the breath, the focus of the poses, the release of trapped feelings, and the energy that yoga poses allow. This abiding calm had an impact on both my prayer and my meditation; it also moved into my life off the mat into my daily activities and relationships.

My investigation into yoga started with the body postures and finding a style that suited me. I eventually found it. Integral *hatha* yoga taught me to feel my insides clearly—to practice something difficult, sometimes physically stressful, but that led to inner peace. Many benefits were immediate. I learned poses that I could take into the workplace to give me a sense of calm and serenity. A simple forward fold into "rag doll," arms hanging limply to the floor with the gaze at the legs, would bring circulation to my brain and both increase alertness and provide a release from anxiety. Calm, measured breathing in a mindful pattern would dissolve anger and fear and return me to the present moment. "Standing mountain"—simply standing in an aligned, balanced manner—would bring composure as well as a sense of strength and valor. All of these activities would remind me that I was sufficient; I was enough in myself and with the universe. Returning to the mat on a regular basis developed, strengthened, and renewed these skills.

Unlike with competitive activities, in yoga I was being taught to explore my physical limits in balance and breath, with love and acceptance for where I was, moment by moment. The philosophy of yoga also intrigued me; my teachers were generous with their time and wisdom. Here, I thought, was another way to look at recovery: with guiding principles, disciplines, and observances that sometimes mirrored, sometimes complemented, and sometimes expanded on what I had been practicing in twelve-step recovery. Both belief systems were founded on the principle of nonharming. In recovery, cessation of the activity or behavior that debilitated you is the first step of nonharming. In life, treating self and others with care and respect is a continuation of that practice. Both systems believe that honesty, open-mindedness, and willingness are keys to a successful journey. Purity or cleanliness—that is, being right with our Higher Power and others—is a daily practice of both yoga and the Fourth Step, as well as the Tenth Step in particular. Finding contentment in daily life can be achieved through gratitude. The discipline of working a daily program of recovery and mindful yoga practice are partners in this journey. Prayer and meditation are integral to both paths, as is working with a teacher or sponsor. Meetings and *satsang,* or wise company, are suggested. Letting go of control, being in acceptance, and having gratitude become parts of everyday life. In both yoga and twelve-step recovery, being of service, or practicing *karma* yoga, is vital to both internal growth and communion with your Higher Power.

I was able to use what I had been learning on the mat—to use the postures with controlled breathing and a focused mind to become more self-aware—in my approach to life and self-discovery, and apply the yoga philosophy to enrich my Eleventh Step prayer and meditation beyond measure. I was truly being "rocketed into" what the Big Book (the basic text) of Alcoholics Anonymous (p. 25) describes as the "Fourth Dimension," one day at a time, one practice at a time, one discovery at a time. Yoga, its roots more than 4,000 years old, helps us to be in life one breath at a time, one pose at a time. The practice and guidance of yoga invite us to leave the ego-self and to discover the essential, authentic self. In recovery, we develop a closer relationship with our Higher Power through a spiritual experience. In yoga, the physical exercises, breath practices, ethical observations, self-discovery, and meditation also lead us into a deeper relationship with the divine. In the practice of both yoga and a twelve-step program we seek to unify the body, mind, and spirit.

I was soon off to the races again, but this time in the enthusiastic pursuit of health. I began studying yoga and yoga philosophy. I became a yoga teacher. I enrolled in workshops and went on retreats to figure out how I could bring the beauty of yoga to those in recovery—those who might also have the curiosity and need that I felt. I am finding more and more people on a similar path, those who love recovery and yoga and who share in the desire to move from the Basic Texts onto the mat and into our true natures.

EXERCISE

FIRST BREATH PRACTICE

Three-Part Yoga Breath *(Dirga Pranayama)*

The three-part breath is an important technique that promotes relaxation and calming of the mind. It is often the first breath practice to learn in yoga. It moves one into mindful breathing. The benefits in healing or balancing the emotions are also great. When the mind is calm, it can also become clearer. In having the ability to relax, an individual lessens the harmful effects of stress on the body.

Focused three-part yogic breath awareness is often practiced while sitting comfortably in a cross-legged position on the floor, or in a straight-backed chair, though it can also be done while lying flat on the back on the floor. Novices may find it easier to learn this breathing technique while lying down, since you can better feel the breath as it moves through your body.

To perform the three-part breath, sit the in the comfortable cross-legged position or in a chair (or lie on your back), and close your eyes. If you're sitting, make sure your spine is straight and erect. Relax your body and face. Start by observing your natural breathing pattern. Allow any distracting thoughts to drift away. Without judgment or attachment, invite them to come back later. Bring your attention back to the breath, allowing your focus to remain on the breathing.

Inhale through your nose, filling the belly with your breath as if it's a balloon; exhale, expelling all breath from your belly through your nose, pulling in the stomach to make sure it's empty of air. Watch that your breathing is smooth and relaxed, without any strain. Repeat several times, and then move on to the next step of this breath practice.

Perform the next inhale like the one before, but when the belly is full of air, breathe in a little more so the air enters the lower chest. Your rib cage should expand. Exhale from the chest first, and then exhale from the belly. Repeat this several times before transitioning to the third and final type of breath in this *pranayama* (breath control practice).

Inhale into the belly, then the lower chest, and then the upper chest so it expands and lifts your collarbones. Exhale through the nose, from the upper chest first, then the lower chest, and then the belly. Continue this for about ten breaths.

Return to your own native, natural breath and continue for a full minute before leaving this practice. Notice how you feel. Your breath is portable! You can use this type of focused, measured breathing anytime. It will add health, vitality, and ease to your life, and it can soothe you in trying situations, bringing patience and well-being to every moment. With time, this can become your conventional breathing pattern.

CHAPTER TWO

What Is Yoga?

THERE ARE MANY DEFINITIONS OF YOGA, all of which depend on the context of what is being presented, especially in Hindu scriptures. There are schools, lineages, and unique practices. There are myriad interpretations of the original writings, with different areas of emphasis. For some, the term *yoga* refers exclusively to the physical practice, but for others the devotional aspects are of equal importance. I am going to keep it simple here and let the more in-depth explanations come later as we delve into our yoga practice.

Essentially, yoga is a philosophy that includes a system of physical postures, mindful breathing, and meditation intended to unify and balance the body, mind, and spirit in order to bring enlightenment, or an understanding of our true nature. In contemporary Western terms, it would lead to the understanding that we are not our ego but our soul, or higher self.

The Bhagavad Gita says, "Do thy work in the peace of Yoga and, free from selfish desires, be not moved in success or in failure. Yoga is evenness of mind—a peace that is ever the same."[1] Or, as Tav Sparks eloquently puts it in his book *The Wide Open Door,* "[Yoga] is the name used in India for the transformation of consciousness. Basically, yoga refers to the yoking, joining together, or union of the individual self with the Divine self, or Higher Power."[2]

The term *Higher Power* as used in recovery is often seen as synonymous with a God of monotheistic religions. That definition works for some and alienates others. The concept of a single God can be incorporated into the practice of yoga. The underlying concept is that we all have a divine aspect within ourselves, within the illusions created by the ego-self. The journey is to remove these illusions to find the true, genuine, authentic self. To generalize, while Western religions search for an external source or authority to aid one in the search for the divine, Eastern religions look inward.

In discovering yoga and its philosophy, I found new ways of expanding this inner journey. I required some tools and methods to penetrate and dissolve the shell of ego, fear, insecurity, and denial that obscured my true nature. Yoga has a broad palette to choose from to help discover one's true self, to reveal the selflessness, compassion, trust, and care in one's core. To achieve this unveiling, there are yogas of devotion, duty, self-study, and physical practices for well-being. These can be incorporated into your life whether you believe in a monotheistic God or you are an adherent of an Eastern religion and are seeking alignment with the divinity within you. Your Higher Power can remain of your own choosing as you expand your tool kit to include additional practices to enhance your journey.

I will introduce several types and styles of yoga that are helpful in expanding recovery work. We are most used to hearing about the physical practice of yoga—the postures or *asanas*. Particularly in the last few decades, many new applications of *hatha* yoga have been designed, developed, and popularized in the West. There are systems and there are schools, and the majority of these focus on the poses; the philosophy is not usually a critical component in the studio or gym.

These styles are all variations of *hatha* yoga, and are developed, redesigned, or focused for a specialized approach to working with the body. The classical forms of yoga reach back to more basic poses performed in a style that focuses on integrating body, mind, and spirit. In that the true purpose of all *hatha* yoga is to unite body, mind, and spirit, to bring union to the entire true nature of a person it is helpful to be less focused on developing the body beautiful. My approach relies on the classical forms and poses and uses them in the furtherance of the original purpose—to "yoke" or bring together all aspects of ourselves—in the search for balance and peace for those in recovery. It is important to remember the seminal purpose of the *hatha* yoga practice: to bring oneself into balance in order to find union with the true inner core of one's being. It is to prepare the body to be comfortable to sit in meditation. (See appendix I for a list of some more popular styles and lineages of practice.)

TYPES OF YOGA

The major types of yoga include *mantra* yoga, *bhakti* yoga, *jnana* yoga, *karma* yoga, and *raja* yoga. *Hatha* yoga is a part of *raja* yoga.

MANTRA YOGA

Mantra (**mahn**-truh) yoga uses sound or phrases as a meditation tool. The focus on a sound or phrase can bring the mind to stillness. It is also the yoga of sound and sound repetition. A specific word or phrase, often designed or assigned to a student by a teacher, is repeated in the mind both during meditation and throughout the day. It is not only the meaning of the words, but the actual sounds of the syllables that are believed to have power. The sounds and vibrations of the words, spoken silently or out loud, are likely to bring about powerful transformation: unity with the divine. Negative self-talk can poison our self-image and growth. Replacing this toxic mind-noise with a *mantra* can be very beneficial for those in recovery.

Words said to us as children, offhand comments tossed out in an unthinking manner by a relative or family friend, can reverberate their untruths in our minds throughout our life. Addicts can often perpetuate these "*mantras*" with our own pejorative phrases: "You are too (fat, stupid, lazy)," "You are not worth (saving, good health, escaping abuse or danger, having love, receiving compassion)," and so on. Repeating these phrases over and over can become a script, a self-fulfilling prophecy for our lives. Replacing these toxic repetitions with healthful *mantras* is the key to "right thinking."

I used to refer to myself as "stupid" constantly. I would drop a pencil, and I was stupid; I would be late for an appointment, and I was stupid; I made a wrong turn while driving, and I was stupid. How foolish and harmful! I changed it to "silly," from *Winnie the Pooh,* many years ago, and that has made a tremendous difference over time. It allowed me to refer to myself in kindness, with the hope that I would learn and grow, but with an understanding that this is how I am NOW. Working on the deeper habits of negative self-talk came from this revelation, and I have been able to change many other habits of thinking, resulting in a positive change in my outlook and an increase in self-acceptance.

What would you say if I told you this practice of *mantra* yoga is used in the rooms of recovery? It's true: we use slogans and prayers in our daily lives to get us through difficult times and alter our reactions to situations; yoga made a science of it thousands of years ago.

BHAKTI YOGA

Bhakti (**bak**-tee) yoga directs attention to our emotional natures, our passion, and our love, and dedicates these aspects of ourselves to our spiritual quest and union with the divine. The compassion and affection that all those in recovery feel for one another, which we hear about at meetings, is an aspect of devotional yoga. We search for that true relationship with our Higher Power, our inner being, in this quest. Coming to the realization that we can hold our Higher Power, our divine nature, close to us in every moment of everyday life is a breakthrough that helps recovering people as they work the steps and move toward health.

The yogic style of devotional music known as *kirtan* is a form of *bhakti* yoga. The ancient words of the songs, the call-and-response process of the singing, and the vibrations of the voices and instruments truly bring one closer to one's Higher Power. Any form of devotional and inspirational music, such as gospel, classical, or instrumental, among others, can be seen as a yoga utilizing all our passions and directing them in a healthy and reverent manner. The various prayers recited at meetings and the choral readings of the Twelve Steps can be interpreted as a form of *bhakti* yoga; we are listening to our highest desires for ourselves, and through this repetition we align ourselves with our Higher Power and right thinking.

JNANA YOGA

Trying to discern the real from the unreal through the use of mental faculties is the practice of *jnana* (**jan**-ya) yoga. Using insight, knowledge, and wisdom, we search for the true self; *jnana* yoga leads us to our true self by removing all that is not our true self, or our false beliefs. This form of yoga relies primarily on the intellect.

Referring to the work of Tav Sparks, the study of *jnana* yoga and working the steps go hand in hand. *Jnana* yoga involves using our will "aligned with the Divine Will" and the skills of "discrimination, renunciation, the cultivation of our spiritual impulse" as well as "tranquility, self-restraint, abstention, endurance, concentration and faith."[3] The use of these tools underscores the fact that we must practice our program with a sponsor or another mentor in addition to practicing yoga, and thereby incorporate these yogic skills in the process of working the steps. The Twelve Steps take us through a process that is very similar to *jnana* yoga.

Once we have surrendered our addictive behavior and have established or developed a spiritual path, we begin looking at our deluded thinking. We evaluate our past behavior and try to see the themes and trends in our thinking and past values. From that point we work with our sponsor to get outside wisdom on what we are beginning to discern as modes of unwise, unuseful thinking. We use this process to "disrobe reality to find the divinity within." Throughout recovery we return again and again to this process of thorough review as we become more and more perceptive about our behavior and motivations, both past and present. For ongoing issues we practice Step Ten, taking a daily inventory of both the good and the bad, the useful and the unhelpful, gaining insight and knowledge from that process. By practicing these principles we move toward integration with our authentic self.

Control of the senses and desires through the discipline of self-study can help achieve this union with the *atman*, or self.

KARMA YOGA

Karma yoga is the yoga of action and consequence. Action can be positive or negative. Good (positive) action can come from a clear space in the heart and be performed with no desire for recognition. This type of pure action can be thought of as action performed in dedication to the divine or Higher Power; the action itself is a channeling of the divine and the result is dedicated to the divine. There is no thought or condition of a personal benefit or reflection of that action. *The Bhagavad Gita*, the ancient Sanskrit text in which *karma* yoga is defined and discussed, states that "without concern for results, perform the necessary action: surrendering all attachments, accomplish life's highest good." This is the perfect definition of service: doing what is required and letting go of the results. This is a yogic way and it is the twelve-step way. In the programs of recovery, we perform service to the group by participating in meetings, doing hospital and institution (H & I) work, chairing, acting as secretary, or taking other vital positions, and we perform service to one another by speaking, sharing, sponsoring, and being sponsored. These activities keep us aligned with right action. Many of these do have the outcome of keeping us sober as well as keeping the organization thriving and vibrant. These are not the results for which we do these things; they are the outcomes.

Good action can also come from a well-meaning heart but may have some residual essence of self-seeking or reward. While the action is good, the motives are not as clear or "clean" as those of selfless service. Good or positive consequences may occur, but they are possibly not as beneficial as those of the purest actions. If we do a service for other than a pure motive, it does not bring us closer to our divine self or Higher Power. If I chair a meeting so that I can be known as "Ms. Recovery," and I wish to get acknowledgment or praise for my participation, my good service may indeed benefit others; however, I do not receive as much of a spiritual benefit, as the action is taken to feed my ego. If it was not an offering to my Higher Power or the internal eternal divine, but to me instead, it lacks purity. If I chair a meeting exclusively to be a channel of recovery in action, to be the voice of the Twelve Steps, then I have performed an activity in pure *karma* action.

RAJA YOGA

Raja yoga is also known as the royal yoga, or yoga of kings. *Raja* yoga was designed to bring the body, spirit, and mind into balance so that one can exist in peace and experience well-being. The path of *raja* yoga works with the body, mind, and spirit so that one would find ease in the practice of meditation. It was this integral form of yoga that drew me into its practice, that invited me onto the path of deeper self-discovery, and it is the path I have been following for many years. It is the practice of *raja* yoga in combination with the Twelve Steps that has brought me to a more profound level of recovery. It deepened my inner journey of self-acceptance, of right living, and of recovery of body, mind, and spirit. These benefits and my belief in the relapse-prevention value of *raja* yoga brought me to write this book and is its major focus.

Raja yoga was codified in writing for the first time by an ancient Indian sage, Patanjali, in the form of verses known as *sutras*. These verses documented the physical, emotional, mental, and spiritual steps that would lead to enlightenment: knowledge of our true selves. This is that part of us that is free from the disturbances of the ego and the confusion of self-centered thinking, speech, and action. Enlightenment comes as we know the innermost self, the divine center, our *atman*. There are eight limbs on this path that progressively lead to greater and greater degrees of integration. While these steps are sequential, they are not exclusive; one builds upon the other and each is repeated many times, just like those in a twelve-step program.

SANSKRIT TERMS

The original language of yoga is Sanskrit. The words used to identify the "eight limbs of *raja* yoga" are most commonly referred to by their Sanskrit names. While these terms are strange sounding, they are pronounced fairly phonetically. They are part of the parlance in many yoga magazines, texts, and some classes. Their use is not to alienate the "uninitiated" but to preserve and honor parts of this ancient tradition. To become familiar with these terms, I offer them to you here. The eight limbs are the *yamas* (restraints), the *niyamas* (observances), *hatha* (the physical yoga practice), *pranayama* (breath control), *pratyahara* (withdrawal of the senses to the internal landscape), *dharana* (concentration), *dhyana* (meditation), and *samadhi* (super-conscious state, union with the universe).

The restraints (*yamas*) are five activities we refrain from performing. The observances (*niyamas*) are five activities we attempt to incorporate into our daily lives. In summary, the eight limbs are:

ENGLISH EQUIVALENT	SANSKRIT TERM
The Don'ts—Restraints	The *Yamas*
The Dos—Observances	The *Niyamas*
Body Control	*Hatha/Asana*
Breath Control	*Pranayama*
Detachment	*Pratyahara*
Concentration	*Dharana*
Meditation	*Dhyana*
Enlightenment—Pure Consciousness	*Samadhi*

We practice nonharming, nonlying, nonstealing, nonexcess, and nonattachment of the *yamas* in our daily life. We also incorporate the *niyamas* of cleanliness, contentment, discipline, self-study, and surrender. Further along we add attention to our physical health and breath. We learn to clear our minds and concentrate, and also to meditate. The result of these practices is gaining *samadhi*, a close relationship with our Higher Power, our spiritual awakening, and our "spiritual experience," and we use "these principles in all our affairs."

Learning about the guiding principles of *raja* yoga may feel familiar to those active in a recovery program. Many of these suggestions are similar to those of twelve-step programs. They are also similar to the teachings from other spiritual or religious belief systems, both Eastern and Western. The philosophy of yoga reframes and strengthens the ethics we are incorporating into our lives as part of our recovery. We are seeking union with our Higher Power, with the divine inside and out.

The various types of yoga can support multiple aspects of a program of recovery. Every yoga practice leads to an enlightening process or discipline that enhances and is enhanced by the Twelve Steps. As we practice the principles of a recovery program in our daily lives, so, too, the daily practice of yoga "yokes" us to a path leading to our true selves.

OTHER SCHOOLS OF YOGA

There are many traditions and lineages of yoga with unique names. They all embrace one or more practices of the other types of yoga to varying extents in defining and creating their unique teachings. Some of these are *yantra*, *tantra*, *kriya*, and *kundalini* yogas. *Yantra* yoga is a Himalayan/Tibetan discipline that employs defined and rigorous breath work which, in combination with rhythmic *asana* practice and meditation, brings one to a higher state of consciousness. *Tantra* yoga focuses on the energies and energetic paths in the body. The yoga practices utilize these energy resources to effect spiritual liberation and rebirth. *Kriya* yoga uses extensive breath practices combined with a study of astrology and other cosmologies to bring about liberation of the self; its adherents maintain that it can provide liberation from one's addiction. Under the guidance of a certified or realized master, a student of *kundalini* yoga uses practices from the other types of yoga to increase self-knowledge, intuition, and higher consciousness. There are other lineages and heritages of this centuries-old practice; finding one that fits with your own needs, curiosity, and character is a uniquely personal quest.

EXERCISE

Author's note regarding hatha yoga: *In the practice of any style of yoga, it is strongly suggested that you seek a well-qualified teacher to instruct you. This will benefit you in many ways: your postures will be properly modified for you to achieve maximum benefit, the discipline of a regular practice with proper sequencing will be enhanced, and you will discover a yoga community that will reinforce and inform your journey.*

JOINT AND GLAND RELEASES

Joint and gland movement and rotations promote release of trapped energy or tension and increase healthy circulation. Movement of the joints and glands in an intentional way each day brings the body and mind into union. Maintaining flexibility in the joints will rejuvenate the body and support a *hatha* practice.

MOVEMENT OF THE FEET, LEGS, HANDS, ARMS, NECK, AND HEAD

* Take up a supported *dandasana,* or staff, position (sitting with legs outstretched and arms on the floor in line with hips).

* Toe bending (flexing and spreading toes to maximum capacity)—ten times per foot. Ankle bending (pointing and flexing foot)—ten times per foot.

* Ankle rotation—ten times per foot in each direction.

* Bend one knee and support the leg with hand under the thigh just above the knee.

* Pull knee to chest, straighten leg to the air, lower it straight to the ground with the support of the hands and arms, and begin again. Do ten times per side.

* Sit in any comfortable, sustainable position with back straight.

* Stretch fingers wide and then clench into a fist in a slow, smooth fashion—ten times per hand.

* Flex and contract each wrist with intention—ten times each hand.

* Make a loose fist and rotate each wrist ten times in each direction.

* Elbow bending—with arms outstretched, bend one arm to touch fingertips to the opposite shoulder. Return to a straight arm.

Repeat with the other arm. Alternate ten times, then bend both arms together ten times.

* Head and neck movements—while seated in an upright position, on an exhale bring the chin to the chest. On an inhale return the head upright. Exhale and stretch the chin toward the ceiling, elongating the throat rather than dropping the head back. Inhale to upright position. Repeat chin to chest, then chin to ceiling, ten times.

* On an exhale, turn the chin to the right shoulder, inhale to center, exhale chin toward the left shoulder, inhale to center. Repeat ten times.

* On an exhale, slowly lower the right ear to the right shoulder, inhaling to center.

* Exhale, moving the left ear to the left shoulder, and inhale to center. Repeat side to side ten times.

Sit in stillness for several minutes.

ASANA

Standing practice for full body movement, incorporating the breath.

"One Hundred Breaths Before Breakfast" Sequence

This is a daily exercise that you can do when you first get up—it can take between seven and fifteen minutes. It can also be done at any time during the day. Pose details are given at the end of the book. Before you begin this or any other practice, take a moment to set an intention—a wish or prayer for yourself. This is conventionally a long-term goal or aspiration such as developing patience, self-acceptance, compassion, or gratitude. Find something that suits you and incorporate that into your breath and movement.

* *Tadasana* (standing mountain) See Appendix III for this and all pose details. Get centered, bringing the folded hands in front of the heart. Breathe four rounds of full, three-part *dirga* breaths.

* Heart opening. Arms stretch wide on the inhale, ease head back, looking up if comfortable. Return to prayer position, hands before heart; gaze down on the exhale. Repeat ten times.

* Hands go above head in upward salute on the inhale; exhale into forward fold. Keep knees bent and soft for the first few times. Do this ten times and end with arms overhead.

* Left arm returns to the side. Exhale arching to the left, right hand extended overhead, inhale to upright ten times. Right arm returns to the side; left arm extends overhead; exhale, arching to the right; inhale to upright ten times.

* Bring hands to waist. Inhale and exhale smoothly while twisting from side to side rhythmically, sixteen times total.

* Right leg back, preparing for warrior II: inhale left arm forward, right arm back, both arms parallel to the ground. Bend left knee to ninety degrees on the exhale, straighten left knee on the inhale and drop right arm to right thigh. Exhale, looking back to right ankle, stretching the left arm up to the ceiling and then back, reaching the body back to the right leg in reverse warrior. Inhale and come up to arms parallel to floor, both legs straight, gazing forward. Repeat, moving between warrior II and reverse warrior ten full breath cycles.

* Legs return to *tadasana*. Repeat for left side, bringing left leg back and lifting the right arm forward. Continue for ten full breath cycles.

* Right leg back, preparing for warrior I: inhale arms forward and up overhead, bending left knee to ninety degrees. Exhale and straighten left leg, folding forward into pyramid pose, bringing

arms forward reaching for knee, shin, ankle, or foot. Each successive time, arch back in warrior I with more intention and fold forward in pyramid pose with more vigor. Do this ten times. Repeat for left side ten times.

* Return to *tadasana*. Give yourself a few centering breaths in this pose. Recall your intention and lie in *sivasana*/corpse pose for a few minutes or more.

CHAPTER TWO NOTES

[1] *The Bhagavad Gita*, translated by Laurie L. Patton. London, Penguin Books, 2008, verse 2.48.

[2] Sparks, Tav. *The Wide Open Door: The Twelve Steps, Spiritual Tradition, and the New Psychology*. Center City, MN: Hazelden Educational Materials, 1993, p. 158.

[3] Ibid., p. 161.

[4] *Bhagavad Gita: A New Translation*, translated by Stephen Mitchell. New York: Three Rivers Press, 2000, p. 65, verse 3.19.

CHAPTER THREE

What Is Addiction?

THERE ARE TWO QUESTIONS HERE: WHAT is addiction, and why do we become addicted? I would like to address the second question before I delve into the first. There are genetic tendencies, rearing conditions, and the emotional/spiritual makeup of each individual. One can have had a perfect childhood with healthy parents, with no history of addiction in close family members, or one can have had an upbringing in a toxically dysfunctional home. There is not one certain path to addiction, but there are commonalities among addicts in how they perceive and process the world.

I believe that I moved down the path to addiction as an aversion to inner turmoil and psychic pain. Why did I allow myself to break the rules (of which I had been inordinately fond as a youth) to hang out with the forbidden people and do forbidden things? Why was I so attracted to risk and danger? My early family life left me with no trust in people, places, and things; trust in these could let you down. Chaos was a constant. I knew from the news, television, and my distressed junior high teachers that drinking and drugs were illegal and dangerous. I had attended Alateen (a twelve-step program for the children of alcoholics) when my mother first attempted to get sober. I was aware of the dangers of addiction, yet the release provided by drugs and alcohol—the complete distraction from daily life—was too alluring to avoid.

My descent into full-on addiction was swift, but it took many years before I finally hit bottom. At first I gave little thought to my feelings of misery, loneliness, and despair. I never questioned these feelings. I considered them to be an uncomfortable part of life that deserved no more or less attention than anything else. When I started getting loaded on a regular basis, I found relief from these painful and terrifying emotions. This was a double bonus! Simultaneously I had found freedom from the pain of life along with the exciting social aspects of drug use and drinking—the music and sex.

I was still very young when I determined that I could not live without these crutches—the booze, the drugs, and the partners. It kept me totally diverted from my pain until I couldn't keep that lifestyle up any more. I was "sick and tired of being sick and tired"; I was unable to keep a semblance of a regular life, and no matter how much I used, I was still in agony. I found that point of no return long before I was actually able to quit drinking, using, and carousing. I came to that moment over and over—still unable to stop—adding self-loathing and a sense of entrapment to my other disowned feelings. My entire consciousness had moved away from searching for my true self, but this true self was pining for life. This cycle lasted until the day I sat on my bed, feeling that the essence of my inner self was slipping away. Not until then had I realized the true nature of this crisis. That was the moment in which I felt I had to make a choice—to walk out of the house and down the street into complete oblivion, or to change, to put down the booze, the drugs, and even "the guy," and to start down the road to recovery. I chose to change. I had had my spiritual awakening.

ADDICTION STEMS FROM A "SPIRITUAL MALADY"

The terms *spiritual awakening* and *spiritual experience* are used in the Basic Texts of twelve-step recovery to describe a psychic change in an addicted person that is strong enough to bring about a change in behavior over time; in other words, a change in thinking sufficient to effect recovery (*Alcoholics Anonymous*, p. 128).

The success of the twelve-step program of recovery in treating addiction is due to the fact that all three aspects of the person— body, mind, and spirit—are addressed. However, the Twelve Steps, in my opinion, don't go far enough in addressing the physical recovery needed. There are also more tools available to investigate the mind, and to nurture the spiritual self. These parts of the journey can be addressed individually in many ways, but I believe, and have proven to my own satisfaction, that yoga addresses all three with precision, compassion, unity, and ease. Of course, millions of people around the world have found recovery in the Twelve Steps *without* the addition of yoga; however, for me, integrating yoga practice into my twelve-step "design for living" is just a natural and very welcome enhancement of my recovery.

For long-term recovery, I've discovered that the spiritual aspects become the most critical. This is a basic tenet of twelve-step recovery: that a well-maintained spiritual life is critical for daily relief from the symptoms of our addiction. What may happen then is that with long-term abstinence, while the physical lure of the substance may be completely gone, the daily life of recovery may have become routine. Meetings and fellowship have become a matter of course, and complacency may have set in. Even with continued enthusiasm for the program, there may be a deeper yearning. This sense of a spiritual craving can occur early in recovery or later on, as it did for me, and when it did it was painful and acute, and it was severe. Reaching for outside help had been a part of my recovery, and it too fell short in addressing the deep-seated pain I was feeling. In spite of the fact that I had continued to be in service, both having a sponsor and sponsoring women, I found myself depleted. I was functioning, but I was uncomfortable in my emotions and body, and I was weary in my heart. This was the point where I hit the skids and found I needed more. This was when yoga entered my life.

Yoga addressed the spiritual craving. It does unite body, mind, and spirit in one fluid practice, so it began to address the disunity I was feeling in my soul. Yoga helped me find a way to explore my internal spirit and combine my sense of that nascent true self with a concept of the divine—my Higher Power. Since then I have practiced yoga regularly, and I believe that yoga is a powerful tool to enhance recovery from the outset and improve defenses against relapse. The sophistication of a yoga practice, the variety and elements it has to offer, allows for it to be introduced to people at different phases of their recovery. This makes yoga a versatile tool for any addict.

Early in recovery the physical aspects of yoga—breathing, stretching, relaxation, and meditation—can help every day, one day at a time. Mindful breathing reshapes the emotions, and feeds and calms the brain. The yoga postures release tension and stress, allowing trapped energies to be freed, as well as bringing vitality to the entire body. Relaxation techniques can give respite to the addict, giving a total body-and-mind "time out" from the rodent-wheel churning of negative emotions and bad ideas. Finally stepping into the bliss of meditation can teach mental composure. Moving into this state, one can learn about the habits of the mind and how to become detached from them—taking the role of the observer. This can be a way to develop self-awareness.

TAKING A STEP BEYOND

There is a stage in recovery I call the "second suffering" in which you realize your separation or alienation from your genuine inner self.

This stage can come at any time during recovery, from the moment your body is detoxified, or later when daily life gives way to the inner longing for completeness. Initially we come to the rooms of recovery expecting only to be relieved of the symptoms of our addiction, or maybe to be taught a way to participate with our addiction in a pleasingly controlled manner. We become disabused of the second idea right away. We soon learn that overcoming the symptoms is a lifelong journey that both confounds us and exceeds our expectations.

There is a process we go through in order to fully address the symptoms of our disease, and one that goes beyond the superficial, technical "get out of jail," "make your way back into her heart," and "get my job back" kinds of activities. The process involves intense self-discovery and finding a power greater than your ego-self. Coming into the rooms of recovery, as countless thousands discover, you "come," "come to," and eventually "come to believe." This state of coming to believe may take the form of finding a connection with a monotheistic religion. It may mean reestablishing yourself in a church, temple, mosque, or other place of worship from your childhood or youth. It may mean coming to terms with a period of suspended belief/disbelief in which you hold your spiritual questions in abeyance while you ride under the wings of the group's faith. Or this can be a time in which you begin your own spiritual journey— your quest to find a spiritual home, your communion with the divine.

The ache of knowing there is an inner self, but the anguish of not knowing what it is, can be overwhelming. It may bring one to the brink of emotional relapse. Whether or not one uses again, the emotions tip back into old ways of thinking, speaking, and acting. Decisions come from old sets of values, and one's "inside" (self) and "outside" (presentation and ego) move away from each other. This results in a deep spiritual dissonance. The inner being begins to thrash about, needing to be known. Action must be taken to address this, or a "slip" may be next. When this "second suffering" shows up, with its need to know one's authentic self, this is when the deeper philosophical aspects of yoga can become important. Yoga, with its four thousand years of exploration about the spiritual suffering of trying to find our true nature, has developed a science for this search.

To address the question "What is addiction?" there are many views. Addiction occurs in the physical body, with the emotions and the spirit. It is the unrelenting desire to continue consuming a substance or behaving in a certain manner despite serious negative consequences. My readings have included the following point of view: that addiction can be the result of genetic traits, brain dysfunctions, psychosocial or behavioral causes, and emotional dependencies that have turned into addictions. Some addictions are born of the pursuit of pleasure or pleasurable sensations, while others are developed in the avoidance of pain. The progression of going from social drinking to alcohol dependence to alcoholism is known to the sufferers, but it is not well understood in medical circles. There is a medical/modern science view of addiction (which is shared by Central Recovery Press) that says addiction is a chronic, progressive, primary brain disease, and then there are the twelve-step recovery, yoga, and *ayurvedic* perspectives.

MODERN MEDICAL MODEL

In one version of the fable "The Blind Men and the Elephant," three blind men decide they would like to discover for themselves what form an elephant has. They come upon an elephant and each man proceeds to touch and interpret the entire beast from his personal experience. One determines from the tail that the elephant is like a rope. The other, feeling the strong leg, decides the elephant is like a tree. The third, feeling the broad expanse of the side of the body, discovers the elephant to be like a wall. Each is correct about his experience of the part, but they are all restricted from "seeing" the elephant because they do not understand it as a whole. This dilemma can also be faced by the individual practices of classical medicine, psychiatry, and psychology, as each looks at an aspect of addiction and defines it solely from its own point of view. Other, more contemporary approaches use the current clinical addiction model, which defines it as a "biopsychosocial" disease, combining all these points of view.

Alcohol and drugs enhance or interfere with the activity of neurotransmitters and receptors within the synapses of the brain, resulting in a feeling of euphoria or "getting high." Certain activities (viewing pornography, getting lost in a video game, the rush from gambling) can have a similar neurological effect to that of these substances. Some of these effects can have consequences that may remain permanent if the exposure is constant or extreme.

Dopamine is a neurotransmitter, one of those chemicals responsible for transmitting signals between the nerve cells (neurons) of the brain. Also known as the pleasure-sensing chemical, it regulates movement, emotion, cognition, and motivation. The overstimulation of this system, which rewards our natural behaviors, produces the euphoric effects sought by people who abuse drugs and teaches them to repeat the behavior. This dysfunction, this overstimulation of the neurotransmitters can happen in a variety of ways: the neurons transmit too much dopamine, excess dopamine is allowed to transfer rather than being blocked, or the transfer of the dopamine is impaired in total. An increase in the transfer of dopamine—or the balance of this transfer—is created with the use of drugs or with certain stimulating or sedating behaviors. This imbalance in the dopamine levels sets off a process in the brain that destroys the ability to reason, as well as caring and emotional regulation. It also disrupts or destroys memory and intelligence. The euphoric state created becomes desired, and then the need for these unhealthy levels of dopamine, and the addictions that created them, becomes chronic.

The medical model struggles with the treatment of addiction, as there appears to be no single physical cause. The theories and approaches to addressing the symptoms are as varied as the specialties that work with addiction. Addictionologists suggest there may be some chemical deficiency in the brain—part of the neurological system that lets one know he or she is calm, safe, and serene. The chemicals in drugs or alcohol address this lack and provide those sensations. Some psychiatrists suggest that people reach for drugs or behaviors in an attempt to self-soothe during periods of stress. Others posit that the addictive behavior may result from the malfunction of the self-regulation system. The continued need for certain drugs is based actually on the avoidance of the pain and difficulty of withdrawal; this is often the case with nicotine and opiate addiction. According to research done at the Scripps Research Institute, cocaine may subtly change the chemistry of the brain in such a way that the brain begins to release fear and stress chemicals when the user is not taking the drug. These symptoms can be relieved only by ingesting the chemical once again. Thus, having ingested the compound in itself creates a need for the drug.

The medical models are excellent at identifying the physical condition of the addict. The doctors best suited for treating the addict are addictionologists who understand the dangers of exchanging addiction or dependence on one substance or behavior—one manifestation of addiction—for another. They work closely with their patients to move them safely off their primary substance of addiction. Once medical balance has been achieved, referral to a twelve-step program is the next step. Medicine in itself does not "cure" addiction. A comprehensive approach is required.

AYURVEDIC MODEL

Like yoga, *ayurveda* is 3,000 to 5,000 years old. It is a system of healing that focuses on establishing and maintaining balance of the subtle energies within us. It is a complete medical system, based on restoring harmony within the individual as well as between the individual and nature. The basic principle of *ayurveda* is that we are all, at core, perfectly ourselves. We have a natural, basic, healthy balance to our mind, body, and spirit. This natural perfect balance is our home base. This is a critical concept in *ayurveda*, the practices of which are designed to bring us home, home into our divine selves. It is not practiced with a "one-size-fits-all" concept of human beings, but understands that there are different energies that manifest in and influence different people in different ways. These energies are known as *doshas*. One's energies, or *doshas*, can become out of balance, particularly when the body is exposed repeatedly to toxic substances and behaviors. This out-of-balance condition reveals itself in digestion, sleep patterns, immune-response systems, and the look of the skin, hair, eyes, and tongue. Bringing these systems back to balance returns us to our true nature. The skills of an *ayurvedic* specialist can be employed to "heal the fragmentation and disorder of the mind-body complex and restore wholeness and harmony" (National Institute of Ayurvedic Medicine).[1]

Ayurveda describes addiction as "forgetting your true nature." Whatever the manifestation of addiction, when the true self becomes eroded by that disease, the entire being becomes out of balance and symptoms develop. Insomnia, constipation, dry skin, and sinus infections, for example, are called to the attention of the specialist. In his book *Ayurveda*, Robert Svoboda states that the goal of *ayurvedic* medicine "concentrates on inducing right relationship of body with mind and spirit."[2] Addiction assaults this right relationship as we overuse or overconsume, and self-gratification takes over. Svoboda further states, "Each of our addictions . . . is another nail in the coffin of our freedom. True enjoyment (of the pleasures of life) is only possible when there is true health."[3] He goes on to describe the effect of addiction on the brain. "Though substances have differences in their powers to addict, all addictions are fundamentally identical . . . mediated by similar chemical changes in the brain."[4]

Ayurvedic medicine has continued to evolve in its holistic approach to health in order to cope with modern needs and scientific approaches. There is now a specialty known as *sangakara chikitsa* to address the treatment of addictions. This form of *ayurveda* focuses on the dietary, physical, and emotional challenges facing a person in recovery.

According to one of the *ayurvedic* texts, the first and foremost cause of illness is the loss of faith in the divine. This idea is also a seminal part of twelve-step recovery literature; integrated long-term recovery includes a transforming spiritual experience. Incorporating the spiritual self informs and influences the recovery of the emotional, physical, and mental parts of one's being. The spiritual path must be considered as part of a complete plan of recovery.

YOGIC MODEL

Yoga understands the negative mental tendencies that exist in humans. They are called a "misperception" in the yogic texts. This includes the "misperception of the impermanent as permanent" and the "unconscious for the conscious," among other misleading mental constructs. The Sanskrit term for this is *avidya,* and it is believed that misperception is the root cause of all human suffering and the main impediment to achieving peace of mind. What could be more misleading than believing there is comfort in addiction? The temporary respite from the deep psychic pain that addictive behavior conceals will eventually give way to more grief and suffering created by the activity.

Habits of the mind manifest themselves in habits of behavior. Reaching for a pill, fix, drink, lover, hand of cards, or another website can be habits of behavior that are self-destructive and are poor solutions for our problems. Yoga describes habits of the mind as *samskara*. These are types of ruts or grooves in our thought patterns. By bringing our attention to them and by practicing new thinking patterns and initiating new behaviors, we can create new and healthy *samskaras*.

Yoga teaches us that there are five layers, or *koshas*, to the human being. There is the physical layer; the energy layer; the thinking, feeling, and sense layer; the values, discerning, or intellectual layer; and finally the emotional layer, which has the potential for sustained joy. The first two refer to the body, the second two refer to the mind, and the last refers to the spirit. Ultimately, all five layers are a covering for the seed of the transcendent, authentic, core self—the *atman*. These layers are interconnected, each having an influence and effect on another or others. This explains how a disease of the body will affect the mind and spirit, an impairment of the emotions can have an effect on the spirit and body, and so on. Another way to understand these layers is to understand what fuels and sustains them. The physical layer is nourished by food; the energy layer is nourished by breath; the senses and thinking layer is sustained by the mind; the values and intellectual layer is enriched through intelligence and wisdom; and finally, the emotional layer is nourished with joy and well-being. Understanding the five layers or *koshas*, which sheathe, conceal, and protect the transcendent self, and understanding the interconnected nature of the sheaths help us to see the complex benefits of embarking on a holistic road to recovery.

Yoga gives us a fourfold approach to creating and improving health: (1) identify the symptoms, (2) discover the cause, (3) establish a goal, and (4) choose the best tools to obtain the desired result. Following these steps provides a framework for healing the body, mind, and spirit. You may note that this approach is not so different from Western medicine. You see a doctor with a specific complaint, a diagnosis is obtained, and a treatment plan is developed. The difference is in the identified relationship between symptoms and causes as well as the healing tools used by the various approaches to health and wholeness.

In recovery programs, the first three of the Twelve Steps identify the problem, a factor in the cause, and a goal in finding true health. The rest of the steps are, to a larger extent, what is needed in terms of tools. However, the Twelve Steps primarily address the intellect and core values, in addition to establishing a spiritual path and developing an abiding relationship with a Higher Power. Addiction had created a condition of living with false values and developing strong mental schemes of denial, defensiveness, and rationalization. These bloomed into full-fledged delusion when it came to understanding our own affliction of addiction. Using the steps to clear the path for the goal—a life of recovery—was vital in terms of defining how we used the steps, the tools, to create and improve health. A sustained recovery path, however, requires a more complete and integrated approach and includes the health of the physical body.

Addressing the addiction and its afflictions, we may find a need also to address the physical body beyond abstention. In yoga this includes the energy body, and a manner of living that brings us into union with the kernel of the innermost self. We use healthy eating and physical yoga practices (*asanas*) to heal the physical body. We use breath practices to heal the energetic body. The guides to proper ethics and values in relationship within us and with others help heal the mind. The self-awareness that is developed in the yoga practice, along with having worked the Twelve Steps, allows us to heal the emotions. In moving toward emotional healing we may find a reacquaintance with an understanding of our true spirit. A holistic approach to healing body, mind, and spirit is then the set of tools that we reach for in treating addiction, and yoga can provide these tools. Combined with a twelve-step program as a foundation for recovery, yoga complements, expands, and incorporates the wisdom of that program.

Whatever the manifestation of addiction, yoga, with its holistic approach to wellness, will address the unmet needs of the spirit, mind, and body. This ancient tradition has the answer to the suffering of life—tested through the ages and available to everyone who wants to utilize it. This is both the entryway and the foundation of all yoga practices.

TWELVE-STEP MODEL

The twelve-step definition of addiction has been cited above. It covers the disease in all its forms: mental, spiritual, and physical. The steps are some of the first tools to be found in identifying the disease and its cause, and they provide instructions for a process necessary to peel away old behaviors and find self-awareness. This self-awareness is critical to developing the skill and discernment to acquire new values and levels of compassion and respect for self and others.

Compassion and respect become cornerstones for new behaviors, which lead one to deeper and deeper communion with one's Higher Power. Working with a sponsor helps with marking progress toward the goal of being one's better, true self. Initially upon entering the rooms of recovery, we wanted only one thing—to be released from the obsession to gamble, take drugs, smoke, buy goods, or whatever the harmful behavior was. We wanted to stop. We did not consider that we would also improve, grow, and blossom as human beings. That was far from our minds.

More than once we have heard in the rooms of recovery, "If I had made a list of what I wanted my life to be in recovery, I would have sold myself short at every turn." By that we mean that we had no idea so much would change, or that we would have such an improvement in our quality of life. Once that becomes apparent and some of the healing begins, the initial goal changes to one of living life more fully. Once a degree of self-awareness is achieved, it may become clear that more may be needed than what can be found in the rooms of recovery. This is where yoga and the health and self-enlightenment attributes and teachings it offers are a natural fit. At any rate, this is what I have found.

Some addicts first address their disease in a medical office, others in the office of a psychologist, psychiatrist, or other mental health professional, and some through the demands of the courts. Some people reach out to their spiritual advisors to embark upon their path to recovery. Nearly every case will be referred to a twelve-step program. All roads do lead to a path that urges a threefold approach to addressing the disease: physical, emotional, and spiritual. Yoga takes them all into account, and it does so completely, on all levels including the subtle spiritual levels, and it reintegrates the body, mind, and spirit in a way no other path is able to accomplish.

It does not matter how or when you discovered your addiction or "how far down the scale you have gone," yoga can rehabilitate you. As I recently learned, the words *sanity*, *health*, and *wholeness* are interrelated, the root of one leading to the next. These three words—from the books of recovery and yoga texts—address body, mind, and spirit in the union of health, and they help establish us in our true selves. This is particularly true on the path of recovery. Yoga can restore sanity and health and bring us to wholeness.

EXERCISE

ASANA

"One Hundred Breaths Before Breakfast" Repeated

Take a moment to set an intention—a wish or prayer for yourself. This is conventionally a long-term goal or aspiration such as developing patience, self-acceptance, compassion, or gratitude. Find something that suits you and incorporate that into your breath and movement.

* *Tadasana*—standing mountain. Get centered, bringing the folded hands in front of the heart. Breathe four rounds of full, three-part *dirga* breaths.

* Heart opening. Stretch arms wide on the inhale, ease head back, looking up if it is comfortable. Return to prayer position, hands before heart; gaze down on the exhale. Repeat ten times.

* Hands go above head in upward salute on the inhale; exhale into forward fold. Keep knees bent and soft for the first few times. Do this ten times, and end with arms overhead.

* Left arm returns to the side, exhale arching to the left, right hand extended overhead; inhale to upright ten times. Right arm returns to the side, left arm extends overhead; exhale, arching to the right; inhale to upright ten times.

* Bring hands to waist—inhale and exhale smoothly while twisting from side to side rhythmically, sixteen times total.

* Right leg back, preparing for warrior II: inhale, left arm forward, right arm back, both arms parallel to the ground. Bend left knee to ninety degrees on the exhale, straighten left knee on the inhale, and drop right arm to right thigh. Exhale, looking back to right ankle, stretching the left arm up to the ceiling and then back,

reaching the body back to the right leg in reverse warrior. Inhale and come up to arms parallel to floor, both legs straight, gazing forward. Repeat, moving between warrior II and reverse warrior for ten full breath cycles.

* Legs return to *tadasana*. Repeat for left side, bringing left leg back and lifting the right arm forward. Continue for ten full breath cycles.

* Right leg back, preparing for warrior I: inhale, arms forward and up overhead, bending left knee to ninety degrees. Exhale and straighten left leg, folding forward into pyramid pose, bringing arms forward and reaching for knee, shin, ankle, or foot. Each successive time, arch back in warrior I with more intention and fold forward in pyramid pose with more vigor. Do this ten times. Repeat for left side ten times.

* Return to *tadasana*. Give yourself a few centering breaths in this pose. Recall your intention and lie in *sivasana*/corpse pose for a few minutes or more.

CHAPTER THREE NOTES

[1] Gerson, Scott. *Basic Principles of Ayurveda* [Online]. Available from http://www.niam.com (accessed 15 June 2010).

[2] Svoboda, Robert V. *Prakriti*, Second Edition. Twin Lakes, WI: Lotus Press, 2010, p. 4.

[3] Ibid., p. 6.

[4] Ibid., p. 7.

CHAPTER FOUR

Combining Yoga and the Twelve Steps of Recovery

HOW DID I COME TO INTEGRATE yoga with my recovery program? Once I had started practicing yoga, I came to wonder how I could *not* combine the two. With every new discovery about the practice and philosophy of yoga, I felt an internal reverberation of recognition—nearly a sense of déjà vu. I repeatedly told myself, "I recognize that." I seemed to have some inner reference that made this all seem so familiar. The *yamas* and the *niyamas* felt like a natural fit with the ethics of recovery; several types of yogas espoused beliefs and practices that extended my nascent skills in these areas. When I met a "friend of Bill's" who was also a yoga student, she had the same feeling that this was a path that we knew. While taking classes together, we would just look at each other and smile in agreement when something familiar was covered.

The similarity begins with the rooms of recovery, which are magical places. As someone has said, "They are a miracle of disorganized organization." There are no recovery policemen who go around ensuring that meetings are run according to the "approved form." We do have the Twelve Traditions that each group follows with care. The meetings are self-monitoring and comply with basic rules of order, with some variation as to style and focus. Even without official supervising monitors, the traditions of that particular recovery group are usually followed and the service needs of the organization are met. Recovery meetings are peer-led; there is no single leader—the process is shared. There are common books, a special language, and traditional ways of imparting information, both at a group level in meetings and one-on-one with a sponsor (a program guide). Anywhere you go in the world, the format of a meeting will be similar and the message will be the same: "You don't have to use anymore. Welcome. We care." Each new member is embraced with similar enthusiasm wherever meetings are held. This is the invitation, and the newly recovering person is always the most important person in the room. The message is: "The struggle is over if you want it to be."

Yoga studios, too, can be havens from the madness of everyday life. Walk in and remove your shoes (as you symbolically leave behind the concerns of your daily life); roll out your mat, take a seat, and breathe. Center and prepare yourself for the meditation side of the practice and the turning inward. While recovery meetings follow a very similar format from location to location, yoga classes, too, generally follow a similar structure. That is where the similarity ends. Each yoga class and style includes varying amounts of philosophy and spiritual references. This is where attention to your personal journey comes in. You will practice discernment in selecting a style, studio, and teacher or teachers who will help you grow in the direction you desire.

Beyond the physical practice, however, yoga will lead to peace. Yoga, in its centuries-old wisdom, offers an end to suffering—being separate from your authentic self. It does this with an invitation to pursue a path of unity, bringing body, mind, and spirit together in the quest to find your awakened self. The similarities between yoga and the original twelve-step programs is not an accident. Bill Wilson was a student of Eastern religions. He was also a follower of Carl Jung, himself a student of these ancient philosophies. The influence of these beliefs may account for the feelings of there being a similarity between the program of recovery and the various yogas expressed by those I have met who practice both.

Due to the rise in the popularity of yoga, it is now much easier to find a teacher than it has been in the past. Taking the time to find a studio that suits you and finding a teacher or teachers who support your journey will prove invaluable. Incorporating your recovery program work with your yoga class will make the experience on the mat much more powerful. But make no mistake—attending recovery meetings on a regular basis is crucial for sustained recovery. While a consistent *hatha* (physical) yoga practice will enhance your recovery, no one ever relapsed from missing a few yoga sessions. Missing twelve-step meetings, however, is generally considered a major ingredient in the recipe for relapse. My yoga practice is an invaluable component of my own personal recovery, but I know that for recovery from the deadly disease of addiction, steady participation in the program of recovery is critical; *hatha* yoga practice is not. Meetings, working with others, and developing healthy relationships with sponsors and those you sponsor will save you from a deadly disease. However, the principles of yoga will sustain and aid you in your journey to self-realization, which may be as crucial for you as it was for me to prevent a relapse.

FINDING THE BLEND—YOGA AND RECOVERY

In your quest for a deeper understanding of the history and teachings of yoga, there are texts widely available, from the *sutras* of Patanjali to the *Bhagavad Gita* in its lovely translation by Stephen Mitchell. There are beautiful books with pictures of poses and wonderful volumes describing the various yogas, yoga styles, and the individual limbs on the eight-limbed path of *raja* yoga. There are groups and schools that offer classes to investigate these writings in depth. However, there is a challenge when you want to understand the yoga philosophy from a recovery perspective. At present, there is a growing trend of new groups and meetings being formed that combine the two; reaching out through Internet search browsers will uncover them. These organizations and events provide a structure for discussion and a group of like-minded people with whom to meet, network, and study.

My introduction to the deeper philosophical offerings of yoga occurred when I studied to become a yoga teacher. I embarked on this rigorous training in order to get a guided education. I pursued my studies with a classical teaching program rather than a more physical yoga-based school, specifically so that I would be able to teach people in recovery. This investigation has proven to be never-ending. I obtained a knowledge of the basics in that training program and have continued to read and take training courses in order to broaden my base of knowledge. I also learn from the curiosity of my students as I continue to teach. The ongoing response I have received from people who have found that this yoga practice greatly helps their recovery has made all the work worthwhile.

Introducing yoga to people in recovery is a beautiful process. The first step is overcoming their belief that one has to be flexible to practice yoga. In fact, the only flexibility needed is a mental one. I have brought yoga classes to the incarcerated, to the recently released in halfway houses, and to a variety of studios and retreat centers, and I also conduct private, one-on-one sessions. In each class we begin with the breath, set an intention, and share a nugget of yoga philosophy, and then move into the *hatha* practice. After our poses, moving from standing to sitting to lying-down postures, we conclude with a period of relaxation. Occasionally this is coupled with a guided meditation. We close the class with a remembrance of our intention and a moment of gratitude, and we share the phrase "*Namaste:* the light in me dwells in the light in you; the good in me honors the good in you." The mindfulness of the breathing, the concentration brought to the poses, and the release of tension during final relaxation are a gift to experience and observe. A woman who has been studying with me for nearly two years had this to say: "Having now practiced weekly for a period of time, I am now beginning to understand yoga's eight limbs as a way of life . . . a lifelong journey of spiritual growth." Another student, a nineteen-year-old man, said, "When I get tense during the day, I can stop for a minute and breathe, and then I know everything is going to be all right." This is how a guided yoga class for people in recovery can feel to students of all ages and abilities.

Investigating the similarity between the recovery program and yoga, finding parallels in their respective practices and literature, allows one to thread the two paths together. The recovery program philosophies are found both in the approved literature and in the informal sources of key ideas and suggestions. Some of the program foundations are expressed through the aphorisms or sayings that are displayed in many places, from meeting-hall walls to bumper stickers.

We utilize only those approved sources as references in meetings and other public forums. They are the official guides. One of the powerful admonitions and sources of counsel in recovery is the acronym HALT, which stands for Hungry, Angry, Lonely, and Tired. When hungry, angry, lonely, or tired, we are more prone to a "slip," a return to our addictive substance or behavior.

So, too, yoga teaches us to be mindful of our physical and emotional conditions. We are advised to eat wisely in both a physically and emotionally nourishing manner, being mindful of the food and its properties and source as well as the flavor, and of our well-being as we eat. In twelve-step programs, we are cautioned to avoid being hungry, and to learn to take care of ourselves in a routine and careful manner. The anger part of HALT is addressed in the principles of recovery (for instance, love, tolerance, restraint of tongue and pen) as well as in yoga. Those of us with addiction can no longer luxuriate in the intoxicating and exciting feelings of anger, for this extreme has been found to be toxic to us. In the observance of yoga, we find that anger is harmful—in thought, word, or deed—and that these feelings are not useful to our life of enlightenment and our path of self-discovery.

Yoga is also a community. In *ashrams*, or yoga centers, it is a little easier to identify that community. In a yoga studio or class, we have to listen more carefully to find those who practice a full yogic life—beyond the physical practice of *asana* or postures, to include a moral life of nonharm to self and others. Yoga encourages us to find community (*sangha/satsang*), the wise company of other aspirants with whom to share intellectual and spiritual growth. This is similar to the dictum of recovery programs to find the healthy ones in the pack. In recovery we are urged to maintain closeness with the "winners" in the program—those who stay close to the principles and meetings. It is suggested that we do not become isolated with our thoughts and our own company. This aloneness could become loneliness, and this can be dangerous. We cannot afford to get too lonely. In the yoga community we find those who share similar interests and seek them out. Perhaps a yoga teacher can become a mentor, a person with experience and disposition who can provide a place, guidance, and time for insight and discovery.

YOGA AND SELF-DISCOVERY

As we move into recovery, we find that we had not taken adequate care of ourselves at any level. The cycle of addiction and addictive behavior disturbs the rhythms of our lives. We eat poorly and isolate ourselves, but we also do not sleep well. It can take quite a while to find a sleep pattern that refreshes us. As an example, I had always thought that I was a night person. It came as quite a surprise that I really function better in the mornings, and I must get a good night's sleep by going to bed earlier than when I was using or even in my early recovery. With its attention on controlled, cleansing, and nurturing breath practices, yoga can help you sleep better. *Hatha* yoga, the physical practices, can release trapped energies and tensions that tend to make the mind run on. A regular routine of *hatha* yoga promotes regenerating rest. *Yoga nidra* is a process of total physical, mental, and psychic relaxation. It is most often practiced with a teacher who guides you through levels of the detachment of awareness into a very restful state that is not yet sleep. Regular practice of *yoga nidra* can benefit the body and the mind, promoting mental clarity. Using yoga as a recovery tool can help one avoid becoming too tired. The various practices of yoga can enhance the tools that we regularly use on our path of recovery.

The Twelve Steps provide a supported way to peel the onion of the self in security and with intention. There is an elegance in beginning the healing process by asking for help and placing oneself in the care of a beneficent being—our Higher Power. Feeling safe in this care is critically important for the next step of the process: being able to rigorously assess both the perceptions of our life up to this moment and our actions in life events. We are asked to look at what has distressed and destroyed us in our lives, and how we have violated our intuitive ethics or morals in creating and coping with these events. We could not do this alone. We needed to rely on the care of our Higher Power as we went through this process, as well as on the loving, accepting ear of a sponsor or mentor.

Yoga shows us that our Higher Power is actually an aspect of our greater selves and that every experience, even the negative addiction, was created by us to lead us back to our true self. Once we have identified and accepted all parts of ourselves, we can be more fully receptive to the promises of twelve-step recovery, leaving guilt and self-recrimination behind us in the process. As we discovered the themes of our transgressions (fear, greed, insecurity, anger, and so on), we could then reflect on the power they have had in our lives and examine the ways we have responded to them.

Using the guidelines of yoga and the steps of the program, we will be better able to change our behavior by discovering our habitual responses. Identifying the habits of our nature that no longer work, we can investigate the root causes. Their removal comes by turning them over to our Higher Power—not by living in denial of these character challenges, but by being willing to have them taken from us. So even these negative feelings, thoughts, and behaviors become teachers leading us to our true selves. After we mended our harms to others in the best way we knew how, we continued to be mindful of our impact on others in our daily lives. Having cleaned the slate to a great degree, we are now able to sit in meditation and move closer to our Higher Power and embrace it as an aspect of our greater self. Ultimately we will bring ourselves—these new, clean, and aware selves—to the service of others.

WORKING THE STEPS "YOGICALLY"

Investigating the form and interpretation of one's Higher Power is an intensely personal experience. Each person finds his or her own resistance and then peace with this discovery. Yoga is not a religion, and it does not have a "God." Whatever your religion, yoga can help clear your body, mind, and spirit so you can better appreciate and participate in it. In yoga, the idea of a Higher Power is actually the true spirit that is resident in our true, authentic selves. This self (or soul) is part of the universe of selves. The philosophy of yoga is that one's journey is to remove all the layers of the ego (the self-seeking and self-centeredness we talk about in recovery) to find the true self. Having embraced the Twelve Steps of the recovery program, moving to "practice the principles in all [my] affairs," "letting go," "surrendering to win," and being in service, one may still find oneself at an impasse at some point.

Even in recovery one can feel "restless, irritable, and discontented." As I grew in the program, I continued to be impatient with my defects of character and shortcomings, and I harbored a hard heart toward myself. This lack of self-forgiveness and self-love was having an impact on my ability to develop healthy self-esteem. I felt I was a failure at "doing the program"—participating adequately in the twelve-step program. I blamed myself for not going to enough meetings, not working with others as much as I should, and not relying properly on my Higher Power; you name it. Even though I continued my therapy, I was stuck. Others saw a goodness in me I didn't see, nor did I believe was there. On one hand, I knew there was a greater purpose, or reason, to my life and my growth; on the other hand, I was afraid that I was a sham and that others might be fooled, but I certainly wasn't. I was not worthy. The problem was that I hadn't yet integrated my Higher Power into my *self*, had not yet accepted the divinity inside me, in my heart, at my core. There had to be another way to find the me I wanted to be, the me I was told was at my core. This took a whole other process of peeling my way in and down, of trust and self-study, of practice and eventually meditation. In my search, yoga provided me with the way.

The *samskaras*, or tendencies, created during our active addiction are areas that also must be healed. Those habits of self-deprecation and self-aggrandizement, the guilts and shames, the remembrances of harms done and harms received, all need to be healed at a deep level. We don't want to stay stuck in the past or live in regret of past actions taken and not taken; we must find a way to remove the slippery mudslides to self-abasement that these ruts can provide. With the use of the Twelve Steps and the traditions and the guidance of yoga and meditation, we can heal ourselves at that deep level, resist following these negative *samskaras*, and create new, healthy habits of mind to enable us to live closer to our Higher Power, and in a state of ease.

The practice of yoga is a way to deepen your practice of the Eleventh Step used in most recovery programs, which invites us to employ prayer and meditation to become closer to our Higher Power. We seek both guidance and the skills to further our usefulness in the world. Following the philosophical and spiritual teachings of yoga and the physical *hatha* practice leads one inside oneself. The attention to the breath and body is centering and focusing; the *sutras*, discussion of them with teachers, and reading of the works of the luminaries who have interpreted and written from these texts give rise to deeper thoughts and investigations into the true self. Yoga, like the Twelve Steps, is a "practice." There is a progression of actions to take in order to move yoga into one's life, just as the practice of the steps, over the years, becomes a natural way of being in life. Day by day, bit by bit, it becomes part of your life. For those in recovery, it is like coming home for the second time.

Another similarity between the philosophies is that recovery programs, whether they call it this or not, make use of *mantra* yoga, which is a science of sound and its healing effects that goes back thousands of years. We say opening and closing prayers, and we have readings that become choral recitations in some meetings, so familiar are the phrases. It is not uncommon to hear people say that they had been chanting the Serenity Prayer "like a mantra" in times of difficulty or challenge. Yoga practitioners discovered that this activity is an effective way to quiet the mind, move out of the ego and its emotional self-talk, and align with one's higher self or Higher Power. We say this prayer and other phrases over and over so that the very rhythm and sounds have meaning and evoke a feeling of calm and safety. Phrases and affirmations, aphorisms and prayers, can also be brought into *asana* practice and repeated to bring focus to the mind and heart and alignment between all aspects of the self.

Bhakti yoga, the yoga of devotion to one's Higher Power, is practiced when we recite the various prayers together, listening to our voices speak in union of what we hope to embrace as a group and in support of one another. Each recovery program has favorite step-related prayers that are read in meetings or recited on one's own that invite the best of our selves to be in union with our Higher Power. We ask that the less useful attributes of ourselves be removed in order for us to be of maximum service to others. We practice *bhakti* yoga when we turn our will and our lives over to the care of our Higher Power. The experience of devotion can also be found in the passionate adherence to a life of recovery, in order to be a person living the values and gaining the insights to fulfill our true purpose as human beings. Whether on the mat or the meditation cushion, in the meeting rooms of recovery or with our sponsor focusing our concentration on hope and gratitude, these practices bring us in union with the divine in an expression of *bhakti* yoga.

Steps Four, Six, and Seven are all parts of self-study—removing the unreal to reveal the genuine. This is a type of *jnana* yoga, to move us closer to the divinity within, and it takes a lot of effort. A speaker I heard at a conference described it like this: "To a newcomer, we old-timers look like ducks floating on the surface of a pond. What you don't see is that we are paddling like hell underneath." This unpeeling of the layers of illusion and delusion is a constant practice of self-study that continues throughout our recovery as we meet additional challenges in life, and as we move through the stages in our own life. In this process we come back to our own essence, to who we are, how we act, what we contribute, and how we handle our fears, insecurities, anger, and other negative emotions. How, too, do we deal with excitement, opportunity, and growth? We have to study our reactions and responses and reacquaint ourselves with this new "me."

Karma yoga is the yoga of action and its natural consequences— good and bad, intentional and unintentional. The consequences of our actions may be local, in our family, community, or country; or they may have distant effects, like when we purchase goods made with slave labor halfway around the planet, thus perpetuating that tragedy. By becoming aware of the interrelatedness of all our actions, we become more and more cognizant of ourselves as part of the web of existence. None of us bounces on this trampoline of Earth without affecting another being. This is not a judgment but rather an observation. We are aware of this in recovery, referring to this process with the phrase "In order to keep it (recovery), you have to give it away." Working with others is one sure way to stay in recovery. Being of service to others is what we are ultimately called to do in recovery. Being in recovery ourselves, in and of itself, can be a beacon. As we also say, "You may be the only Big Book/Basic Text that person has ever seen." This means that you and your actions speak for recovery wherever you go.

We participate in the spiritual aspects of yoga when we "let go and let God," when we perform a service, or when we do "the next right thing," as are suggested in the rooms and the Basic Texts of the twelve-step programs. We practice getting out of our own way, letting go of our egos, and giving the results to God. As *karma* teaches us, to every action there is a consequence, and for people in the "action of recovery," the result is a better life—not a life free of life, but a life you get to live on your own. "Nothing is so bad that using won't make it worse." This is a mantra we live by—a phrase we repeat to ourselves when the perceived pain of our outlook and illusion-based mind makes the action of drinking or using seem like an option. We also hear in the program to "think the drink/drug through"—look at the consequences of that action and then decide not to use. The Tenth Step gives us a moment each day to reflect on the outcomes of our actions, to see where the natural *karma* of consequence has come to pass. Practicing *karma* yoga mindfully is a way to deepen the practice of recovery—by being totally aware of the consequences of our actions.

As people in recovery, whether from debt and consumerism or unhealthy sexual relations, food, or drugs, we are also yogis practicing *mantra, bhakti, jnana, karma,* and *raja* yogas, just by following the principles of our twelve-step program. The search now is to learn more about the nuances of these yogas and bring them more fully and mindfully into your life, to help find your genuine inner being—the true source of your solace.

The path of *raja* yoga was the path chosen here to move into a higher state of self-awareness, self-acceptance, and self-love. It is the yoga practice that has most helped my own recovery and that of my students, as I have refined its application over the years. The eight limbs of *raja* yoga do not line up with the Twelve Steps in the same progression; however, they do weave and dance through and with one another in a beautiful blend of inner harmony. The progression of this book will be to follow the eight limbs of *raja* yoga and to "feather in" the steps and other wisdom of the twelve-step programs. We will also investigate the *gunas* and *doshas* and use these ancient *vedic* concepts of the physical and emotional body as diagnostic tools and paths to recovery and relapse prevention.

EXERCISE

TWO-TO-ONE BREATH PRACTICE

* Taking the tall-seated position on a chair or the floor, become aware of the posture, the length of the spine, and the softness of the facial muscles, relaxing the shoulders and the collarbones. Bring the mind to consciousness of the breath, in and out through the nose. Investigate first the length, depth, and duration of your breath right now.

* With consciousness, move into a deeper breath by extending the inhale. Allow the exhale to be of an equal duration. Repeat this

several times: breathe in and breathe out—evenly. Count now the duration of the breath—om-one, om-two, om-three, om-four—on inhalation and do the same on exhalation, slowing the breath down. Repeat this three times.

* Now increase the exhale by one count so that the inhale is four counts and the exhale is five counts. Repeat this new pattern three times; inhale for four counts, exhale for five counts.

* Extend the exhale again by one count, to six. Repeat this pattern three times.

* Again extend the exhale by one count, and repeat the four-count inhale, seven-count exhale three times.

* Repeat the increase a final time, coming to a four-count inhale and an eight-count exhale. Repeat three times.

* Reverse the progression until the counts of the inhale and exhale are again equal for three rounds. Return then to your personal breath duration and depth. Sit in stillness for several minutes.

The following is a simple visualization exercise that explains much about our practice. Many yoga teachers use this story; many yoga students may recognize it. I paraphrase it here:

Imagine a carriage, pulled by horses, carrying a driver and a passenger.

> The carriage represents the body.
>
> The horses pulling the carriage represent the emotions.
>
> The driver is the mind.
>
> The passenger is the soul.

The story goes on to say that the state of the average person is as follows:

The carriage is in terrible disrepair.

The horses are half-wild.

The driver is unfocused and drunk.

The passenger is asleep.

Yoga, it is said,

Repairs the carriage (body),

Tames the horses (emotions),

Sobers and focuses the driver (mind),

And reawakens the passenger (soul).

This is the purpose of yoga.

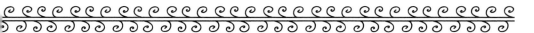

CHAPTER FIVE

The Yamas

THE *YAMAS* ARE THE RESTRAINTS, OR guidelines, we use to refine our relationships with our communities and ourselves. As Deborah Adele says, "Yoga's guidelines do not limit us from living, but rather they begin to open life up to us more and more fully."[1] When we follow these tenets, they lead us away from wrong thinking, destructive actions, and behaviors that cause suffering. Unenlightened actions and behaviors occlude our eternal internal selves from being free and shining through us. When we abide by these codes, we become one with ourselves and partake in the provident grace of the universe.

AHIMSA, SATYA, ASTEYA, BRAHMACHARYA, AND APARIGRAHA (Nonharming, Nonlying, Nonstealing, Nonexcess, Nonattachment/-clinging)

Ahimsa: Nonharming. In the *sutras* of Patanjali (2.30), he emphasizes "consideration for all living things." He goes further and states (2.34) that "a sudden desire to act harshly or encourage or approve of harsh actions can be contained by reflecting on the harmful consequences." We start the journey of *raja* yoga with the guideline of nonharming. *Ahimsa* is the first *yama* (restraint). I don't believe it was an accident that Patanjali began the yoga *sutras* with nonharming. (As you may recall, the *sutras* document the physical, emotional, mental, and spiritual steps that lead to enlightenment: knowledge of our true selves.) This concept of *ahimsa* remains the basis of every restraint, observance, and limb on the path of a yogi, and it is also integral to the path of recovery. It starts with how we treat ourselves and expands to how we treat others. This is a back-and-forth dance that can also move from noticing how we affect those around us, back into our thoughts and deeds to see how we treat ourselves. Each step teaches us discernment about what is harmful and what is neutral. It is also based on the yoga concept that we are all one, and what we do to another we do to ourselves, and vice versa.

Yoga philosophy underscores the importance of thought by emphasizing the impact of intention. T K V Desikachar writes that the *yamas* are more "attitudes and behaviors"[2] than restraints. He suggests that one's true intention is the seed from which one's behavior blossoms. As thought guides actions, the flow of intention and energy (*prana*) also determines where our enlightenment develops. Unpeeling the layers of the ego helps us discover the real self. In yoga, this real self is in union with all other real selves. As we become more sensitive to the impact of negative thoughts and behaviors, we can see that this kinder attitude results in perceiving a kinder world. When anxious, angry, or resentful, we see this in our attitude and behavior with others. A dark and cloudy emotional interior manifests itself in a stormy relationship with others. Harm to one is harm to all.

Often harmful thoughts or actions can arise from a feeling of powerlessness. Reading one of my favorite books, *The Yamas and*

Niyamas by Deborah Adele, I was heartened by the way she addresses powerlessness. Feelings of powerlessness are a big issue for those in recovery. While we acknowledge that we are powerless over our addiction, many of us have to find a sense of balance and control in our lives in general. She states, "Feeling powerless leads to outward aggression in the form of frustration and anger, or withdrawal inward into depression and victimization."[3] She further suggests that nonviolence is not an embracing of powerlessness but engagement in a feeling of competence by facing your fears—all of them, large and small. She encourages a mental shift, moving away from feeling powerless in three ways. The first is moving into gratitude—trusting in the moment and thinking about others. This is in line with the twelve-step programs as we "maintain an attitude of gratitude," stay in the moment, and are of use to our fellow man. The second is reevaluating certain stories we have about others and ourselves. Do they still apply? The last way is developing skills, as is heard in meetings, "to meet life on life's terms."

Ever mindful of how I address myself in my head, how I treat myself throughout the day, and what I expect of myself in the day and beyond, I need to remember this restraint. In truth, once I had gone through the steps of recovery, I found that I really did have to treat myself as I would others, in addition to treating others as I would my best self. When I come from my best self, my healthiest self, I treat others with kindness, patience, and understanding. When I am not hungry, angry, lonely, or tired (returning again and again to the HALT of the program), or restless, irritable, or discontented, I am more conscious of the impact of my behavior on others. I am more sensitive to the negative effects of my less-than-wonderful characteristics upon them. When I am coming from my genuine good, I am mindful of being overgenerous with my advice, overhelping others, and getting in the way of their own journey. This intrusion into the life and life path of another can also be a form of harming. We can do harm to ourselves by being critical and judgmental with our unreasonable expectations and negative self-talk. We can do harm to others by jumping into their lives and taking away their ownership of their own paths with an excess of advice and assistance. We can harm both others and ourselves with negativity or invasiveness.

How to practice *ahimsa*, nonharming, can be illustrated by the way we behave on the mat. Learning from the physical practice, we can also see our approach to life. A brisk, vibrant practice may represent a brisk, energetic activity level through the day. Pushing limits on the mat may illustrate a certain striving in one's personal life. Pulling back and avoiding full participation in our practice can also inform us; it can be an indication that we are not participating fully in our off-the-mat lives. These observations advise us when practicing the third limb of yoga—*hatha* yoga—to be mindful of *ahimsa*. When stepping on the mat, be watchful. Watch your practice. Become aware of how you approach, hold, and release the *asanas*—the postures. Consciously remark to yourself how you rest and integrate poses, what you are aware of between the postures. How can we bring *ahimsa*, nonviolence, to our practice as well as to our life? Recalling that harm can be manifested in thought, word, and action, take this awareness of *ahimsa* and see if it can teach us where and how we might be harming ourselves. "Am I moving too swiftly, too deeply in the poses, am I staying longer than my breath advises? Am I harming myself by only going through the motions—mind wandering, mind cheating myself out of the present moment, the present form or posture? Being mindful of finding that place of balance between effort and ease, how is my practice today? Am I holding back, not giving myself fully and with a conscious mind to my activities? Am I throwing myself too fully into what I do, jam-packing activity into my day and life, leaving no time to savor what I have done or even to savor the moment of not doing?" Take the time to ask yourself these questions and listen to your answers.

Watch and, just for today, don't harm yourself by overreaching, criticizing, or short-changing yourself by not being all you are. Watch yourself, without judging. Watch yourself and learn.

EXERCISE

---

1. I will stop harming myself in my actions by:

2. I will stop harming myself in my thinking by:

3. I will stop harming _____ by:

Satya (nonlying): "Right communication through speech, writings, gesture, and actions" (*sutras* of Patanjali, 2.30). "One who shows a high degree of right communication will not fail" (2.35).

T K V Desikachar goes on to explain that "the ability to be honest in communication with sensitivity, without hurting others, without telling lies and with the necessary reflection requires a very refined state of being."[4] Do not be discouraged! It is practice, not perfection. The intention of leading a life of truthfulness is a journey, and every stumble leads us to a new awareness about our ego-self, something we might not have known had we not employed the refinement of reflection and the intention to be truthful in all we do. When we keep truthfulness as our goal, we may become more alert to those moments when we shade true meaning. With this awareness we cease living in the shadow of the ego-self—that part that "makes up" a truth. This false truth may have been established to paint a more pleasing picture of ourselves that we wished to present. It is no longer comfortable to live in the lie of the false projection. For example, while I merely want to be seen as helpful, I may actually just be meddling in the affairs of others or controlling them. True helpfulness comes from doing what needs to be done quietly and without fanfare or advertisement. True intention speaks softly. The lies we tell will tell on us—"pull down the covers" on what we are trying to conceal. We practice removing all that is not truthful so that we can excavate the illusions of the ego to find our true selves.

As the restraint of *satya*—nonlying or truthfulness—comes after *ahimsa*, we will see that nonharming will be inherent in all that we practice from now on.

I am a person in recovery; I do not poison my body with intoxicants. That reason for my incessant lying is now gone. I used to lie about when I drank or used—how much I consumed, how much money I spent, and whom I spent time with—to allow me to continue to use and drink unabated. But lying was habitual—necessary or not, lying came naturally to me—even after I entered recovery. For example, if I was telling someone how frequently I had gone walking in the prior week, I would exaggerate, saying three or four times when the truth was really two. I wanted them to think better of me, so I lied. This is a defect of mine: wanting the approval of others even when that is based on a lie. Then, of course, the approval means nothing because I know I have presented myself falsely. This is the conundrum of lying. The Twelve Steps invited me to look honestly at my character defects and my moral shortcomings. Lying to others was not my only problem; I also lied to myself.

Honesty is a basic tenet of most recovery programs. It is crucial to excise the liar and prevaricator from our minds if we are to bring our true, genuine self to the new world of our recovering life. This does not mean that we are tactless and mean. It does not mean that we spill our emotional beans with everyone we meet at the first meeting. We develop discernment: When is it appropriate to divulge my recovery? When is it totally imprudent for me to apologize to another for harms done? I would not go up to a previous boyfriend, known for his physical violence, and confess that I was the one who had broken his favorite beer mug. That would not be wise. I could be harmed. I would also not put another person in harm's way by revealing something that would only hurt them. My relief from guilt is not worth an increase in their pain. As moms have been heard to say, "If you can't say something nice, don't say anything at all." Measure consequence and importance and consult another if in doubt. This is not a free pass to "white lie" heaven. It is an opportunity to look to our intentions as well as consequences, sanity, and safety.

In practicing this *yama,* we look at ourselves and our actions and try to be truthful in what we do. On the mat we are to be truthful about our intention, our attention, and our abilities in our yoga practice. In the world we are to be truthful about our intention, our attention, and our abilities in our actions and speech.

In my journey I had to examine the fact that not only must I be honest with others, but I must look at being honest with myself, taking the time to find my own boundaries and my own truth. This took some honest investigation. Again, the research into motives was the key. In the past I had lied to get approval, to have people like me. I felt I had to misrepresent myself to others to compensate for what I felt was a lack in my genuine self. I didn't have boundaries, as I wanted to be all things to all people. I didn't evaluate my actions by using my personal ethics, but by what I thought you would think of me. Once I figured out what my limits, ethics, and intentions were, I could then address them mindfully and act on them honestly. In *The Yamas and Niyamas,* Deborah Adele writes that the truth has weight, but also that it changes. Truth is not static. What was a truth at one phase of our life may not apply in later life. She suggests we "ask ourselves if we are engaged in a truthful pursuit that is right for this time of our lives."[5] In fact, sometimes ritual can move us from one stage to another.

What does this mean in recovery? Addiction and addictive behaviors have just been a coating, a layer between my real, authentic self and my crusty outer shell of ego. Removing the substances and behaviors, however, has not made me ego-free. I must do additional work to remove the illusions of my ego-self to find my true self. The ego is a tenacious beast and will consistently raise its head, wanting me to be seen as something other than what I am. *Satya* causes me to ask time and time again: "What is the TRUTH here? What are my real motivations, insecurities, and concerns?" In the program it means working the steps to find out who I am, making amends when appropriate, engaging the feedback and advice of a sponsor, and working Steps again as the truth in my actions and beliefs reveals itself, and through this process to become real, that is, surrender to my real self.

Welcome to the onion that is *satya* and the support it lends to a wholesome, full life in recovery.

EXERCISES

---

1. Take some time to think, and then write about a time when you were not honest with yourself about your intentions. What was the result?

2. Write about bringing honesty to one of your relationships.

3. For the rest of the day, take time before you act or speak to be certain you are coming from a truthful place.

4. Consider this: What part of you is the liar and what part is always in truth?

Asteya (nonstealing): "Noncovetousness or the ability to resist a desire for that which does not belong to us" (*sutras* of Patanjali, 2.30). He further states, "One who is trustworthy . . . naturally has everyone's confidence" (2.37).

This *yama* is translated both as nonstealing (an action) and as "noncovetousness" (an attitude). At times, feelings of covetousness or the action of stealing may come from a place of deficiency— lack of things, lack of power, and lack of self-worth. There can be complex feelings of scarcity stemming from our youth, our emotional upbringing, or a void in our faith. Practicing *asteya* can be a challenge for those carrying emotional baggage and a lifetime of negative habitual responses. Your ego can cut you off from the bounty of your inner self and from the true knowledge that in and of yourself, you are enough, and more than enough.

The refinement of the difference between the two aspects of *asteya* is that the action springs out of the attitude. In Western culture we give more weight to actions than to the antecedent thought or intention. In the program we talk about honesty and "cash register honesty." We look at the outcome of covetous thought first—stealing—and later begin to delve deeper into the well of incorrect thinking. Once we approach this well, we begin to ponder the incipient thought process.

Nonstealing is so much more complex than just avoiding being a thief. It is the idea of "not taking that which is not freely given." Again, using the subtleties of thought, word, and deed, what could one steal? I stole my own adolescence and young adulthood from myself by my addictive behavior. I stole being a mother from both myself and from my children. I stole people's love and concern for me in my tenacious resolution to put my addiction first. To tell the truth, I was a thief as well, stealing money and goods from others to feed my own habits. Then I quit using and started on the path of recovery. But, as they say, when a lying, cheating, drunken horse thief enters recovery—he or she is still a lying, cheating horse thief! More than just the mode of addiction has to change. *Asteya* asks us to refrain from all forms of stealing; it asks us to consider all manners of stealing and *why* we might be compelled to steal. Manners of stealing include things, of course, but it is also others' time, concern, attention, and opportunity, and also the future of our planet, among other nuances that come to mind. If I finish your sentence, solve your problem, ask your advice with no consideration of taking it; if I overbuy and overtrash, I am taking what is not freely given. Sometimes theft can be of things we covet, or someone's personal point of view or lifestyle. We might want someone else's capability on the mat and hurt ourselves by overdoing it. We might feel entitled to more than we get at work and steal time, accolades, or office supplies. We might steal from the moment by living in the past or the future.

In recovery we are encouraged to dig into ourselves, finding the "exact nature of our wrongs" (*Alcoholics Anonymous*, p. 59) and to make a start on remedying them, making amends, and leaving our shortcomings behind us. When I started practicing yoga, I began to deepen my understanding of the nature of my wrongs, looking not just at the act and outcome, but also to the underlying themes—the lengths to which my ego-self would go in order to present a certain image—to protect my nascent authentic self. I had to reflect on the true reasons for my desires, the defects of character that perpetuated my feelings of scarcity within. When we engage the help of our Higher Power, making use of our growing spirituality in dealing with what we know about ourselves, we can find faith in our core. *Asteya* is another tool we use to look at those finer aspects of stealing and thievery, and to circle back, using our Higher Power, to reflect on the intent of covetousness and use the steps to figure out WHY. Do I feel less than others, so I have to ask for "advice" when I really want attention? Do I steal the limelight to take focus from someone else? Do I desire your pose or practice because I feel bad about my own? The growth away from stealing—the growth toward *asteya*—comes from finding gratitude in one's thoughts, feelings, actions, and ideals. You begin with honoring where you are. This is a critical component. Be who you are, where you are. You then begin developing a plan about how to get to where you wish to go. You let go of the results, but make a plan and follow it to the best of your abilities. If I want something more— skills, rank, acquisitions, or other things—I should work for it! Rather than living with a feeling of entitlement ("It should have been me") or resentment about another's achievements, I should educate myself and learn and practice the skill I covet, rather than stealing from a person or stealing their thunder, reputation, or goods. Whether it is a deeper yoga practice, more grounding in the steps and literature of my twelve-step program, or material goods, I will feel better about myself if I work for it. The program of Narcotics Anonymous explains it further by emphasizing that energy, achievement, and closeness with our Higher Power are achieved by getting up and taking action, developing our own inspiration. As you can hear in the rooms of recovery, you develop self-esteem by doing esteemable acts. No one can do them for you; that is why it is called *self*-esteem. So if we want certain achievements, educational benchmarks, personal possessions, or respect or other acknowledgment, we need to take the actions necessary to acquire them rather than steal them from another.

Stealing by providing solutions to another's problems, stealing his or her right and obligation to find his or her own path, is a very subtle action. It is a balancing act between offering advice and providing solicited advice. There is a balance between speaking your truth and taking action that rightly is the other's. I struggle with this when it comes to my own family. When is helping my children "overhelping"? My gut knows. I have to slow down and listen, but my internal voice knows I am attempting to overtake the other person's life. When I am giving too much advice, when I am forcing my idea of the solution onto another, or when I am more invested in a specific outcome than the other person is, I am overstepping my bounds. By invading the struggle, by taking away his or her challenge, I am stealing his or her growth. I must not steal ownership of my children's future from them. As an active family member, this is always an area that is ripe for investigation for me.

Finally, consider *asteya* with regard to the future of our planet. Be wise in what you do and use, be wise in what you buy, be wise in what you trash and how you dispose of it. We are here temporarily. We have current custody of the planet and its treasures and should be mindful of leaving it a healthy place for future generations. We are "current caretakers in this lineage of past and future lives."[6] Practicing *asteya* can wake you up to your own true values and the opportunities you have to grow.

EXERCISE

---

1. Write about an opportunity you have stolen from yourself by practicing your addiction.

2. Write about an opportunity you have stolen from someone else while practicing your addiction.

3. Do you have a desire for or about someone else's life? Can you access your internal bounty to address this?

Brahmacharya (nonexcess): "Moderation in all our actions" (*sutras* of Patanjali, 2.30). It applies to the concepts of both "too much" and "too little."

Brahmacharya used to be translated as "celibacy" but now is more accurately defined as nonexcess, as it refers to all facets and characteristics of our being. Our *prana*, our internal energies, are to be used for our higher purpose. The sensual pleasures may lure us away from healthy relationships, may confuse and distract us from our goal of enlightenment. In fact, the relationship may become our substitute "Higher Power," which, as Patanjali admonishes, is "immoderate." This has been the case through the ages, which is why *brahmacharya* was often translated as "celibacy." In truth, this *yama* refers to the entirety of a relationship—intimacy on all levels, not just the physical connection.

Brahmacharya also refers to all our passions and our desires. In the economy after the recent financial crisis, we became aware of the excesses we had indulged in over previous years. Consumerism, acquisitions, new things and purchases had over extended our credit. We had houses we could not now afford; we had purchased them possibly thinking we could get even MORE money in a quick sale. Others took money out of their houses to purchase more things than they could really afford. Houses were no longer homes, places to live, but they were get-rich-quick schemes to fast track our personal financial growth. We over purchased goods to such an extent that storage containers became a big item! Can you imagine? We own so much that we have to find new ways of storing it all!

We are now also officially an obese nation (The National Center for Health Statistics; 1/13/2010) with 68 percent of the adult population classified as overweight or obese. We consume food in excess of our energy needs. The whole issue of the unhealthy properties of the food we overconsume is another subject for another day. However, we all now eat more than we need to. Many people spend no time or effort in cooking their own food; speed and perceived simplicity motivate people for fast and previously prepared foods. Quantity and frequency are overwhelming our nutritional needs. WE have become disassociated from our nutritional sources.

"My ego likes to feel important, and it doesn't feel very important when I am resting . . . Besides in this culture of constant activity, there is always so much that needs to be done." Activity; doing, doing, doing is our modern mantra; we are always doing something. The more we have on our "to do" list the better, or the more important we feel. The more impossible our schedules, the more valuable we think we are in this overcommitted society. Free time is a fantasy for most, and when we have it, we don't know what to do with it.

Brahmacharya as related to sex can be a challenge in modern times. Sexual activity has become a watered-down sport that is talked about as freely as gum care—and maybe more attended to. Overindulged-in and under-appreciated sex is a recreation rather than a re-creation. So celibacy is out. Another danger of excess is that overindulgence can be a mask that covers a true need and blocks the spirit. With food, things, sex, and time, we find a way to overuse and justify our excesses. Then to top it all off, if you are an addict, excess has no meaning. As an addict (and in one's less than healthy state), there is NEVER such as thing as too much—so the concept of nonexcess doesn't make sense to us.

There is the recovering self that does not ever want to return to the madness of "too much of a good thing is a good thing," where good is relative—the healthy self that continues to struggle with this limit. In our desire for recovery, *brahmacharya* becomes one of the most mindful and challenging restraints. We work with it daily to prevent addictive behavior from slipping quietly from one substance or behavior to another. A friend of mine wrote an article about being a "Teflon Addict." When one manifestation was identified and dealt with, sliding into the background, another one replaced it. We eat sweets and drink coffee with abandon, particularly in early recovery. I struggle with this myself. When I am not practicing this restraint, I can move from one obsessive behavior to another—with only the activity changing—but the mindless indulgence continuing. I cease all other hobbies while I become consumed in that activity. As a result I keep *brahmacharya* in mind as I invite you to do when working on your recovery and your yoga practice.

As we move through abstinence and to moderation, feelings can evolve that had been hidden by excess. With the help of others and with a sponsor/mentor, the core of the issue can be revealed and resolved. This is the core of step work. Finding the point of enough, the grace of sufficiency, the divine in needing what is and having what is needed—that is the practice. That is the struggle and the reward.

EXERCISES

---

1. Write about an area of your life that feels "cluttered" – mentally or physically.

2. Complete this sentence: I am afraid of losing:

3. How have our relationships changed in recovery?

4. Using the idea of forming relationships that nurture our highest selves who do you have in your life now who helps you in this direction?

Aparigraha: Nonattachment "Nongreediness or the ability to accept only what is appropriate." (Sutras of Patanjali, 2.30) "One who is not greedy is secure. He has time to think deeply. His understanding of himself is complete." (2.39)

This is the yoga philosophy of nonattachment. This yama addresses our attitude about possessions. We can practice nonattachment even though we have possessions; practicing the *yama* of *aparigraha* simply means that we are not attached to, obsessed with, or dependent on them. Our possessions should not possess *us*. That is *aparigraha*.

Deborah Adele takes this further in her discussion about being with family: "How many suitcases full of expectations, tasks plans, resentments, and unforgiven moments was I toting around with me every day?"[7] "Let go and let God": you have heard it in the rooms of recovery, and it is in the ether; it appears on cards, bumper stickers, and stationery. Being attached to the way things are, to the way you want things to be, or to the way things used to be brings only pain. Holding on to the results of actions, feelings, and events, and trying to control outcomes or predict the unfolding of events, will all cause suffering. These attributes of clinging, gripping, and even greed can remove someone from the moment and catapult him or her into a dissatisfying future or tie him or her to the past. One grows when one is vulnerable, open to the new and unexpected, the not yet experienced. The moment is where the true self exists—the ego plans and the ego grips to the past. Yoga advises adopting the restraint of *aparigraha*, or nonattachment.

My journey with failing to practice *aparigraha*, whether it has been in holding on to future outcomes or to past experiences, has always resulted in pain and dissatisfaction. Not living in the moment and not living with gratitude just cause more suffering. This living in attachment can include:

• Desire to have events feel like the "first time," remaining attached to the newness of an experience.

  • Food: taste of a dish I had a long time ago
  • Music: the first time I heard a song
  • Feelings: first love or first time of experience
  • The memory of a great high

- Holding on
  - To a present moment
  - To things
  - To my role (at home, at work, in my self-concept)

- Desires for the future of my children
  - Professionally
  - Personally

By clinging, the only experience I am assured of is pain and failure. By failure I mean that grabbing on to these experiences or illusions is like trying (as songwriter Warren Zevon sang) "to grab a hold of a fistful of rain." It can't be done. On the flipside is the fear that by *not* holding on I am uncaring or acting in a noncaring way. Somehow attachment and gripping have come to represent "connection" or even "love." The truth is that I can love and care without being possessive. I can love without being attached to the outcome, process, manner, or event. When I let compassion and care, gratitude and trust be in my heart, when I do find union with and reliance on my Higher Power, there is no need to grasp or hold on. Life events, like a breeze or a gentle wave, ebb and flow at a proper rate and duration. I need do nothing but breathe.

EXERCISE

---

1. Complete this sentence: I am holding on to _____ because _____.

2. I am afraid to let go because _____.

3. I am willing to let my Higher Power help me when

   _____.

EXERCISES

Ujjai breath practice. If you like, you may continue by adding the *asana* sequence outlined at the end of the book. Before engaging in the *asana* practice, bring your consciousness to your heart, the center of your chest, and set an intention for your practice.

CHAPTER FIVE NOTES

[1] Adele, Deborah. *The Yamas and Niyamas: Exploring Yoga's Ethical Practice*. Duluth, MN: On-Word Bound Books, LLC, 2009, p. 16.

[2] Desikachar, T K V *The Heart of Yoga*. Rochester, VT: Inner Traditions, 1995, p. 98.

[3] Adele, op. cit., p. 27.

[4] Desikachar, op. cit., p. 178.

[5] Adele, op. cit., p. 53.

[6] Ibid., p. 65.

[7] Ibid., p. 83.

[8] Ibid., p. 97.

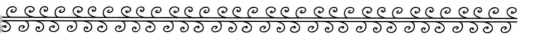

CHAPTER SIX

The Niyamas

THE *NIYAMAS* ARE THE FIVE OBSERVANCES from the second limb of *raja* yoga.

Saucha, santosha, tapas, svadhyaya (swad-hi-ya), and *ishvara pranidhana* are the observances. They translate to Purity, Contentment, Discipline, Self-Study, and Surrender. The *yamas* are our guide in our relationships with others. The *niyamas* are subtle and affect how we are with ourselves at a core level. These tenets encourage us to go deep within ourselves to find that wellspring of truth and authenticity in dealing with ourselves, which has as its outcome greater truth and authenticity when dealing with others.

I think Deborah Adele really captures their essence. "The *niyamas* . . . are an invitation into a radical exploration of possibility. Just how good can you feel? How joyful can your life be?"[1] This joy in life comes from finding our internal bliss, the bliss of discovering the true self, and a constant vigilance to maintain that focus. "The light you seek is within you, so the search is going to be an inward search . . . a journey into inner space."[2]

Saucha: Purity. In the *sutras* of Patanjali, *saucha* is described as "Cleanliness. Or keeping our bodies and our surroundings clean and neat" (2.32). Further, "When cleanliness is developed it reveals what needs to be constantly maintained and what is eternally clean" (2.40). "Dirty clothes make a person look ugly. But they can be changed. If there is dirt deep inside, however, it cannot be changed so easily" (2.41). Beginning with the concept of purity sets the stage for the *niyamas* that follow. This awareness of the mind and its workings will be useful in practicing all the *niyamas*, and, like the waves that move through the Twelve Steps, a further awareness of these observances will curl back and wash over the *yamas* once again. Practicing the latter of the Twelve Steps can bring insights that cause us to revisit the earlier ones. So, too, working the *niyamas* brings relevant awareness to the previous ones. Becoming aware of a cluttered mind, a messy mind, and possibly a mind with the occasional useless or harmful thoughts begins the housecleaning that will be needed to clear a view to a more enlightened future. Tend to *saucha*, and you keep a healthy body and an open, aware mind for all that is yet to come.

Before my recovery, cleanliness, or purity, was not a part of my daily life—neither internal nor external. During periods of hung-over remorse, I would go on a cleaning binge in our house. I would collect laundry, wash dishes, remove garbage, and recycle. I would sweep and dust and bring order to the children's room. In this way I would try to bring order to my life. Many times, however, the garbage would remain stacked at the front door, the laundry sorted in soiled heaps, and the broom abandoned in some corner. So, too, my attempts at self-care would be started with enthusiasm and dropped in despair. A particularly bad morning would find me making all sorts of pledges about drinking and drugs to quit or curtail my use. I would make plans to walk daily, wash daily, to do something with the kids. By four p.m. these dreams too would evaporate with a smoke, a drink, or a line. I certainly couldn't look to the nuances of clean living, much less the outside manifestations of the practice.

Recently I met on a weekly basis with a wonderful group of people to discuss Adele's *The Yamas and Niyamas,* and we shared our experiences as we noted what each restraint or observance meant in our lives. During the weeks we had been exploring the concept of *saucha,* or purity, I found that I had the most difficult time honoring this observance in my life. The difficulty wasn't with the physical aspect—that was straightforward. I had already included many practices such as tongue scraping, using the *neti* pot, and, of course, usual, basic hygiene. I had not been a follower of the advanced practices such as swallowing cotton strips, which are ingested and then pulled out to remove excess mucus in the stomach. I had been practicing physical *saucha:* keeping my person, my possessions, and my house clean. It was the cleanliness of my personal relationships, keeping my side of the street clean, that I found the most challenging. As always, the internal journey was more difficult than the external one. This deeper, more refined practice is a tall order, but with help, I can go through with it! In a twelve-step program we embark upon the action steps to help us "get clean" within ourselves. We begin by taking a thorough moral inventory:

• Working with another to review and hone its purpose, focus, and lesson.

• Coming up with the themes of our broken selves that need attention.

• Reconnecting with our Higher Power in relation to these less-than-lovely parts of ourselves, and asking for and working toward their removal.

• Connecting with people (including ourselves) we have harmed in order to resolve the hurts and harms.

We can then move into a practice of maintaining constant awareness of our actions and repairing damage as it occurs. This action encourages us to honor the finer aspects of our spiritual connections to others, to do right work, and to be of service.

The contemplations in Adele's book ask us to go even deeper into a more subtle understanding of purity. We look into intention as well as action. Yes, we start with the physical body and think about not only the cleansing practices, but also the concept of "garbage in/garbage out." We have to maintain the body in a clean manner by respecting and honoring it by the food we ingest and the drink we pour into ourselves. Further, the concept explores the purity of our relationships between us and our family, our community, and our friends. It is about living a highly accelerated Tenth Step. This requires saying you are sorry not just for rudeness or arrogance, but for inattention and "sins of omission" as well. It applies to mindfulness, not just actions. Holding on to a past moment or living in the anticipation of another "rips off" the present. That is not pure.

I was challenged to find *saucha* in my relationship with some young women. I am a coleader with other yoga teachers in a nonprofit group (the Art of Yoga Project). We bring yoga to incarcerated juvenile females in my county. I had experienced one of those uncomfortable teaching moments when the class was recalcitrant and cooperation low. The girls expressed their reluctance to accept instruction, and the situation began to develop into a confrontation. They were verbally critical and rude about the teaching. I stopped the class and told them that I did not know how to respond to their criticism, or the manner in which it was expressed. We then stood for a moment in silence before proceeding. In the meantime their negative talk escalated, and they were escorted from the room by their regular teacher. In preparation for teaching them the following week, I had to journey inside myself and explore all my various feelings and reactions to their taunting: What were my expectations, and why was I disappointed? What was ego, and what was self-doubt? What was fear, and what was resentment? How do I clear my mind of the past and meet them purely in the moment? How do I remain open to honoring them as they are today, in this class at this time? How can I leave my ego behind safely but provide the boundaries we all require? I reflected on the *niyama* of *saucha* and tried to think about how I would practice this observance and be more mindful in my teaching the next time we met. With my mind and heart clear, the next class was smooth and the present moment was honored. I allowed myself to be confident in the present moment, not allowing my memory of their prior behavior to cause me to modify my presentation. Any lack of participation was allowed to exist within clearly stated boundaries: no cross talk, and questions and comments would be saved for circle time. These would then be seen less as a commentary on my teaching than as a reflection of what that student was feeling. I kept my feelings clean and adhered to my own process; the girls were given the respect of allowing their feelings and actions to belong to them. My fear dissipated, and I was able to be there mentally and emotionally, and not in the prior class.

EXERCISE
---

1. I can find purity in my relationships by _____.

2. I can find purity in my actions by _____.

3. I can find purity in my thoughts by _____.

Santosha: Contentment. The *sutras* of Patanjali state, "The result of contentment is total happiness" (2.42). Finding contentment in our lives applies to all we do, in our homes, in our jobs, and in our attitude as we face life. Contentment is not the same as being resigned, giving in, or giving up. This does not mean a cessation of our labors, but an acceptance of the outcome of our best efforts. To practice *santosha* is to look away from material things, to let go of results, and to quiet the mind. According to *kriya* yoga, *santosha* is a necessary condition for enlightenment, and it paves the way for all that yoga has to offer. In spite of the distractions, perceived inadequacies, or dissatisfactions of modern life, gratitude is the key to reframing our perceptions and finding peace in the moment and contentment in our lives.

Santosha is such a soft-sounding word and an appealing concept. The Sanskrit word itself invites us into its meaning with its sibilant sound—although, like many simple ideas, it is not easy to adopt. To achieve "mental comfort, joy, and satisfaction" we have to overcome future tripping, self-doubt, expectations, ego-ambition, and the need to control others and situations; in general, we need to live in the moment, with full acceptance of what is, and to hold a feeling of gratitude for what happens in our hearts.

While the *yamas* get a lot of press in terms of group discussion, teachings, writings, and understanding, the *niyamas* are discussed and written about less. They are more subtle. Practicing the *yamas* of nonviolence, truthfulness, nonstealing, nonexcess, and nonpossessiveness can have more socially interactive and visible results. The impact of practicing the *niyamas* is highly personal and subjective. Generally, no one will note what you are doing when you practice the *niyamas;* following these principles is more of an inside job. To the discerning practitioner, however, there can be outward effects that affect our relationships. We do not operate in a vacuum; our demeanor, our internal landscape, affects our external interchanges. While we may practice wise speech, even to the point of withholding speech, our facial expressions and nonverbal actions can reveal what we are thinking. The work must first be done on the inside in order to be genuine on the outside—to be seen in visage and in carriage.

What does this mean, and how does it come about? To be content with things as they are does NOT mean that they are swell all the time. It does NOT mean that we have to endure the present, waiting for a more pleasant future. It does NOT mean that we pine for things, people, or situations that would "make me better." We don't even wait for a better, more improved self to enjoy and accept and love our self. In the words of one of the "Ninth Step promises" from the Basic Text of the twelve-step program of AA (*Alcoholics Anonymous*, p. 84), "That feeling of uselessness and self-pity will disappear. We will lose interest in selfish things and gain interest in our fellows. Self-seeking will slip away." Included in this self-seeking are emotional acquisitions as well as material ones: moving toward self-enlightenment and contentment rather than other-focused seeking. Feeling grateful is a vital part of this observance. Finding the good, the beneficent message in everyday occurrences rather than reaching out to other people for the "answer" is part of *santosha*.

The real secret to this *niyama* is letting go of what is not, acknowledging and abiding in what is, with contentment.

EXERCISE

---

1. I find contentment in my thoughts by _____.

2. I find contentment in my surroundings when I _____.

3. I choose contentment in my actions when I _____.

Tapas: Self-discipline. The *sutras* of Patanjali refer to "the removal of impurities in our physical and mental systems through the maintenance of such correct habits as sleep, exercise, nutrition, work and relaxation" (2.32). In this manner, "physical and mental illnesses and disabilities are contained" (2.43). This speaks to the essence of recovery and enlightenment. The shrouding elements of impurities in manners of thinking and illusion can be burned away through the heat of action and transformed. Practicing this discipline on a physical level can lead to detoxification and better health. Following this tenet on a spiritual and emotional level can remove the veils of ego obscuring our true selves.

Tapas is also interpreted as "heat" or "fire," referring to the transformational powers of fire—to change—and also, as in metallurgy, to anneal—to strengthen. Going into the heat of a difficulty, we can resolve a challenge to integrity that results in substantive internal alterations. With the prudent employment of all the other tenets, growth and beneficial conversion can occur. Adele says, "The discipline of *tapas* will mold us into someone of great depth and profoundness if we let it."[3] While one of the classic interpretations of *tapas* was austerity, I find that a more useful understanding of *tapas* is to use what one has to live a modest life, concentrating on developing your person and not your possessions. When we use the preceding *yamas* with *tapas*, the internal focus on discipline and transformation will result in a closer relationship with our authentic seed-self and the divine.

For this recovering addict, self-discipline is and has been critical. When first going to recovery meetings, you may ask, "How long do I have to keep coming to these meetings?" The answer will be "Until you WANT to keep coming." Implicit is the message that you will always keep coming back, working the program so that it works in you.

For me the same has been true when studying and integrating the *yamas* and the *niyamas*. We have to keep working them until they work in us. When I first started going to twelve-step meetings, I would feel lazy or overwhelmed by my life as a single working mother, or angry or resentful at someone at a meeting, or just plain squirrely-brained. I would miss a weekly meeting, then another and another. When I was told that I was missed or asked where I had been, I gave all of the reasons noted above. I was too busy, had too much work, the kids, and keeping up the house and cleaning. "I was resting because I finally had a break or a day off." The excuses were legion. The response from my sponsor and others was often "One reason is a reason, but many reasons are an excuse. There is no excuse for missing a meeting!" This sounds harsh, but I was being goaded into practicing *tapas*: self-discipline. This was the discipline of setting up a healthy habit of showing up at meetings regularly, the discipline of being accountable for my actions, the discipline of taking care of myself.

Now, many years later, I am clear about this part of my *tapas*— meeting attendance—and I have discovered more refined types of discipline to bring into my daily life. There is the discipline of the daily practice of recovery principles, the daily practice of yoga, and daily meditation. All of these seemingly small disciplines ensure that these healthy habits will be ingrained in me in the face of a crisis. In life, there will be crisis: a change of jobs, a change of living space, illness or death of a loved one, illness or injury in myself, relationship changes. All of these could result in a paradigm shift that could cause me to fall off center and out of balance, or even out of recovery.

With healthy habits and disciplines in place, I am more likely to move myself to rights sooner, to find my center and spiritual equanimity with more ease. This is not to say that I am perfect in practicing my daily *tapas*, or to imply that I am perfect in grasping on to the tools that I have at my disposal in terms of support, right action, and looking to my Higher Power. This means only that I grasp them as soon as I "come to" to my need for help, for recovery (in all senses), and for balance. As I can attest, being courageous in this practice can result in phenomenal changes. "Can we stand the heat of being dismantled and changed forever by the fire? . . . Can we stay in the burning [off of our old selves] with integrity?"[4]

Practicing *tapas* means that I have a choice—a choice born of practice—to select the right and healthy way of living rather than succumbing to the addictive ways of the past, the mind cycles and emotional traps that I fell into before I chose to be a person in recovery and a person of yoga.

EXERCISE

---

1. A mental discipline I want to include in my life is:

   _____.

2. A physical discipline I want to include in my life is:

   _____.

3. A spiritual discipline I want to include in my life is:

   _____.

***Svadhyaya*: Self-Study.** The *sutras* of Patanjali refer to "study and the necessity to review and evaluate our progress" (2.32). Beginning with the study of ancient texts to develop enlightenment goals and discernment, we can then move on to examine our selves. While contemplation of our thoughts and ideas is an interesting pastime, we must also involve writings, teaching, and the reflections of others in our ruminations. While the ego may tell you that you know it all, recall where you ended up. The input of others and reading inspirational literature can be very helpful. For those in recovery, it may include the Basic Text of their twelve-step program. Reading texts and not just looking at yourself will also give you a method—a manner or marker—for the ability to "evaluate our progress," as Patanjali suggests. This self-study comes from "true understanding of these [spiritual] truths, which is supported by study of the internal states of consciousness." There is a story told about Michelangelo who, when asked how he came to create such a beautiful statue in *David*, replied that he merely carved away everything that was "not-*David*." So too in *svadhyaya*, we are asked to find the *"David"* or "self" within our own block of marble. There are many layers of protective wrapping that conceal the true *atman*, or self. There are issues—or *karmas*—we are born into (according to those who believe in past lives), those we create with every action, and solutions we find and solutions we take (drugs, food, sex, and things) that conceal our true natures. We hide from ourselves with the roles we take on and with emotions and behaviors (angry coworker, busy mom, or powerful, controlling boss). These are not our genuine inner selves. The work it takes to move toward our inner being can be difficult and painful, but most rewarding in the long run.

In a program of recovery, we are asked to go through the Twelve Steps. Two of these steps require that we first take a moral inventory of ourselves, and then share it with another. With the guidance and feedback from this other person, we can discover the themes of our protective layers. Self-created layers can then be examined. Some layers will be found to be learned "defects of character." We can prepare ourselves for their removal. Other layers were developed out of habits of wrong perception, or of unskilled responses to correctly perceived events—habits that functioned to protect us in some circumstance and are no longer relevant or needed. All of these habits need to be changed, but how? Relying on our spiritual guide, our Higher Power, is critical. This compassionate, loving being will support us during our transition to recovery and its subsequent transformation. For us as human beings, the process is ongoing; we forget, we backslide, and we have to be reenergized along the healing path. Our friends and guides along this same path help and support us. Meetings and recovery friends do this for us. Their journeys can also be reflections of our own, reminding us of where we wish to go.

In yoga, *svadhyaya* also asks us to go deeper to the root cause. To see who and what we really are—spiritual beings having a human experience—is the first step. We examine this outer self or the ego, the fabricated self we present to ourselves and to the world. Before we can make any change, we have to know this ego-self well.

As a teen living in San Francisco, I used public transportation. I would often have to contact the Municipal Transportation Agency (MUNI) to get directions. The operators answered the phone with the following phrase: "Please tell us where you are and where you wish to go." I have held on to that as a given truth: in order to get to a destination, I have to know where I am and also where I am headed. This "finding out where you are" is a critical step in knowing how to get to where you are going (the true self).

Searching for the inner true self requires that we witness, without judging, the present self. This can be achieved by observing how you interact with the world, being aware of what is working to move you along the path to self-realization—and what is keeping you stuck. Observe what is going on in your mind moment to moment; notice what language you use in referring to yourself and others. Is it kind and encouraging, or harsh and critical? What serves to move you along the path? What attributes do you want to foster in yourself to guide your actions with others—control and judgment, or compassion and forgiveness? Meditation can provide moments of silence and practice in moving the mind away from toxic or unhelpful areas. Knowing that you are not your mind, not your body, and not your feelings is a way to conceive of the true self, like Michelangelo's *David* already existing inside of the Carrara marble block that is you. As with that statue, which is more than the rock it is made of, and even more than the art and skill of the sculptor, you too are more than what is seen in this reality. Your true self is inside, waiting to be acknowledged and loved.

EXERCISE

1. A resource for my self-study is _____.

2. A mentor in my journey of self-study is _____.

3. I can rely on _____ to help me in my journey.

Ishvara Pranidhana: Surrender. The *sutras* of Patanjali refer to "reverence to a higher intelligence or the acceptance of our limitations in relation to God, the all-knowing" (2.32).

Many of us have experienced the process and need to surrender over and over; sometimes it is the same issue, sometimes the same subject in a different form. A tool in being able to "turn it over" is to revitalize and align ourselves with our faith, bringing awareness over and over again to the issue, letting go. Our ego, our will, may reassert itself time and time again. This tenacity of the ego to be in charge is the challenge that we face when practicing *ishvara pranidhana*. The more we are able to let go, the closer we are to our divine self and our Higher Power.

Letting go of the results of your work, taking the ego out of them, is part of developing trust and faith in your Higher Power. This is also *ishvara pranidhana*. Clinging to the outcome of our actions forfeits surrender. To give up the outcomes to your Higher Power increases surrender; one can see that both *karma* and *kriya* yogas are embraced in this observance, integrating tenets from other practices. This does not mean to not do your best. Doing what is right with right effort, and then letting go of the outcome or the results, is the very nature of surrender.

This concept and practice comes at the culmination of all the other *yamas* and *niyamas*. It prepares one for the rest of the royal path and for the beauty of the discoveries to come. Be mindful of the ego-self, as it will reassert itself with regularity. Our path is progress, not perfection. It is a practice, and it is the steadfast practice of this *niyama* with the others and the *yamas* before them that will result in a beautiful unveiling of the true self.

Do only that which is before you to do; do not intrude on the work of others. Deborah Adele writes, "As we let go of what we cannot change, we are able to grow more and more into our unique gift and contribution to life. . . . It is an image of strength and softness at the same time . . . to be strong enough to engage each moment with integrity and at the same time to live soft enough to flow with the current of life."⁵

Surrender can be one of the most confusing concepts in the rooms of recovery. We are fighting for our lives in abstaining from our addictive substance or behavior, for it was going to kill us. Then we hear the slogan, "surrender to win." What a paradox!

A lot of preparation has taken place to get here, to this moment in our lives. Working the Twelve Steps of recovery with a sponsor has led to truly seeing ourselves, to seeing who we are and what choices have been made to get us here. It has allowed us to see the patterns we had developed to keep ourselves safe in the world. Working the steps has allowed us to define and identify those character traits and unskilled behaviors that no longer serve us. By our stripping away what was no longer needed, a void was left. I asked myself: if I were not this fearful, yet controlling; shy, yet boisterous; modest, yet uncouth woman, who was I? I was afraid of looking for my true self, afraid of seeing the distasteful, and even more, afraid of seeing the good and the pure. Once a few years in recovery had passed, however, my ability to be aware of myself had stagnated, and my growth had plateaued. I was unable to move closer to the true service of beings who suffer; I was still suffering myself. I felt I did not know my authentic self. My Higher Power and I were no longer close.

I was active in the program: going to meetings, working the steps, meeting with my sponsor, making amends, and working on prayer, meditation, and service to others. You might wonder, as I did, "Is it supposed to be this much work? Who has the time to work on our insides?" But I no longer knew the true me. The woman who stepped into recovery and did the initial work was substantially healthier than the previous one when she was drinking and using. However, it was clear to me after a few years that I was not as well as I could be, and that I was not yet awake and aware. That would take additional work. There is a high cost to NOT going inside, and I was unwilling to gamble my recovery on this chance. So once again—surrender.

So, as the steps moved me through the process of admitting that I am an addict, and further, that I could become healthy, that I did indeed have a Higher Power, and that this Higher Power would support me, I proceeded. I'd followed the suggestions in writing a moral inventory, had shared it with a sponsor, and had done the work of identifying my shortcomings and defects. I became ready to have them removed and walked through the process of making direct amends to those I had harmed. I included myself in these amends and worked at creating a better, healthier life as the act of these amends. I continued to examine my life, behavior, and actions, and remain to this day in constant willingness to be in service and to open myself to the beauty in others and myself.

Finding yoga and working closely with the *yamas* and *niyamas*, as well as the other concepts and guiding principles, has deepened my practice of both the Twelve Steps and my yoga.

True surrendering moves beyond surrendering the control of addiction to our Higher Power. It moves to surrendering our unhealthy behavior patterns to our Higher Power. The act of surrender moves further to surrendering the outcomes of our actions to our Higher Power. Further yet, deep surrender asks that we give ourselves over to the flow of life. Taking the other nine guidelines, the *yamas* and the *niyamas*, utilizing them mindfully in our daily lives, we then are asked to truly surrender, to surrender to the divinity within ourselves.

EXERCISE

---

1. What does surrender mean to you?

2. What feelings or behaviors prevent you from being WITH the moment?

3. What might prevent you from going inside to discover the divine force within yourself?

EXERCISE

NADI SHODHANA—ALTERNATE NOSTRIL BREATHING

How to do it:
For this first practice, use four counts for each step.

* Hold your right hand up and curl your index and middle fingers toward your palm. Place your thumb next to your right nostril and your ring finger and pinky by your left. Close the right nostril by pressing gently against it with your thumb, and inhale through the left nostril. The breath should be slow, steady, and full. Hold for the count of four.

* Now close the left nostril by pressing gently against it with your ring finger and pinky, and open your right nostril by relaxing your thumb and exhale fully with a slow and steady breath. Hold for the count of four.Inhale through the right nostril, close it, hold (four), and then exhale through the left nostril (four).

That's one complete round of *nadi shodhana.*

* Inhale through the left nostril to the count of four.

* Block both nostrils and hold to the count of four.

* Exhale through the right nostril to the count of four.

* Hold the breath outside the body to the count of four.

* Inhale through the right nostril to the count of four.

* Block both nostrils and hold to the count of four.

* Exhale through the left nostril.

Begin with five to ten rounds and add more as you feel ready. Remember to keep your breathing slow, easy, and full.

NOTE: There are many variations of the duration of the inhaling, exhaling, and holds. This is one of many patterns.

CHAPTER SIX NOTES

[1] Adele, Deborah. *The Yamas and Niyamas: Exploring Yoga's Ethical Practice*. Duluth, MN: On-Word Bound Books, LLC, 2009, p. 176.

[2] Osho. *Yoga: The Science of the Soul*. New York: St. Martin's Griffin Press, 2002, p. 91.

[3] Adele, op. cit., p. 144.

[4] Rama, Swami. *The Royal Path: Practical Lessons on Yoga*. Honesdale, PA: The Himalayan Institute Press, 1998, p. 21.

[5] Adele, op. cit., p. 172.

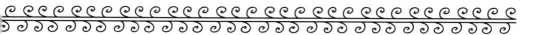

CHAPTER SEVEN

Hatha Yoga

THE PHYSICAL MOVEMENTS OF YOGA ARE themselves an integrative practice. The basic shapes, or poses, are designed with an intention, which is to bring flexibility to the joints and connections in the body, to access energy pathways, and, by bringing the breath into alignment with movement, to focus the mind. Moving in and out of the poses is this intention put into action. This intention, acted upon, helps us obtain certain knowledge and awareness about ourselves. This is the foundation for integration of body, mind, and spirit, and the meaning of the word *yoga:* to yoke or unite. How does the practice of yoga and *hatha* yoga accomplish this? The postures were devised to open the body in specific ways to release and absorb energy. There are poses that aid in the detoxification of the body, opening of the heart, and balancing of the brain. The postures and sequences help move the lymph through the body and increase the efficiency of the immune system. Others help aid digestion and elimination. While not all poses are practiced in every session, over time all the systems of the body are addressed.

The breath is critical to an effective yoga practice. Breath moves oxygen through the body to aid in detoxification and elimination. Ultimately, once the shapes of the poses are learned and the flow from one to the other becomes comfortable, the poses become a meditation in themselves. Focusing on the breath helps us to let go of our thoughts as they come and go, and can bring about spiritual closeness and awakening. Each of these attributes will be discussed at some length in this and the next chapter.

When I first came into a yoga studio with my tight muscles, feeling depressed and full of expectations, I was surprised by how challenging the physical poses could be. As I mentioned, my first teachers were not as in tune with individual needs as my later beloved teachers would prove to be. I did not know there were modifications for poses—adjustments in the pose and the use of props—that could make the pose more available to me within the capacity of my body at that time. When I found a teacher who taught us to practice within our capacity, perhaps at the 80 percent level of effort rather than at or beyond our maximum, the muscle and tension release came. As a person who had experienced much trauma in my life, I had difficult feelings and painful memories trapped in my muscles. I was not only able to tune my physical body, but long-suppressed emotions were also released. Nikki Myers, owner of CitiYoga studio and developer of the Y12SR (Yoga and Twelve Steps of Recovery) class format, says, "The issues live in our tissues." I also found that I did not know how to move through life without being tense. It was usual for me to have my shoulders so tight that they were up by my earlobes. My walking gait was stiff, and my jaw was habitually clenched. I was completely unaware of this tension. Moving into my body, I learned to detect the sensations of tension and relaxation, and that I could choose between them. The poses, and the effort of moving into and out of the poses, allowed me to feel my physical self in a way that aerobics, running, spinning, kickboxing, and other gym-related activities had not touched.

I will talk about the various types of breath practices later, but I must now state how critical smooth, deep, rhythmic breathing is to the *asana*, or pose, practice. I tell my students that the breath will never lie. If the breathing becomes labored or ragged, or stops completely, the *prana* or energy movement of yoga is halted. It signals that you might be working beyond your capacity, or that you have gone into a feeling with such great focus that your vitality is being sacrificed. Take a moment, release the pose a little, or come out of it completely and return when breathing has returned to a deep, slow rhythm. The breath is first and foremost. If all you do for now is mindful breathing, you are helping your body heal. Emotions can block the breath, tension can block the breath, and overreaching can block the breath. Be kind; let the feelings come and let them go. Release the tension and come back into the pose with kindness. The intention of bringing body, mind, and spirit together is harmony.

While *hatha* yoga is the discipline of the body—breath work and the postures help prevent disease and preserve vital energy—it is designed to prepare the body and mind for meditation. Practice of the postures is a physical aid to sitting in stillness, mindfully controlling the limbs and nervous system and preventing them from producing disturbances. The jumpy or lethargic mind has difficulty in coming to the still awareness that is most beneficial in the meditation practice. The uncomfortable, jittery, or blocked body may present challenges when seated in an unmoving position for any length of time. While thoughts leap about in everyone, the habits of the addict's mind are focused on self-abuse, judgment, and negative, unhealthy ways of perceiving the world, and the cycling of those thought patterns can be overwhelming. This repetitive thinking can be even more apparent when we move inside ourselves—either quietly in a *hatha* yoga practice or in meditation. Becoming quiet can let loose some uncomfortable feelings. Looking at them in an unattached manner, breathing through them and letting them go, is a perfect way to practice yoga and your recovery. Tensions, trapped energy, and emotions in the body can be calmed with regular pose practice. With consistency, *hatha* yoga can prepare us for and lead us to a richer experience of the Eleventh Step of recovery: "Step Eleven: Sought through prayer and meditation to improve our conscious contact with God as we understood Him, praying only for knowledge of His will for us and the power to carry that out."

STEPPING ONTO THE MAT

Attending a yoga class for the first time can be daunting. The surroundings and the protocol are new. The mix of athletics and the spiritual can vary from studio to studio, so you might not know what to expect: Is this a studio or class that favors the gymnastics and physical challenge, or is this one that might make you uncomfortable with Sanskrit names and terms? Might this one include chanting and singing to which you are not accustomed? Is it a mix? As a beginner you can try an Introduction to Yoga class or series that will have students who are all at the same level and all learning the practice, the policies, and the precepts at the same time. Or you might start by stepping into an ongoing mixed-level class. Observing other students and how they respond to the teacher is an appropriate way to determine how to behave in a class. However, if you have practiced yoga before and feel more physically adept, you might look for a class or studio that also focuses on spiritual and emotional aspects.

In any of those cases, when you look around to other people for a sense of what is "okay" in a yoga class, do so mindful of your intentions. Are you learning protocol, or are you taking inventory or making evaluations? Looking at the outfit, physique, perceived comfort, or abilities of other students in a type of "echolocation" of appropriateness may be a first step toward judging yourself by the looks of others. Caution must be taken to avoid "moving off the mat" by "judging your insides by other people's outsides" and moving away from your own practice and journey of self-discovery. If you find yourself taking this mental path, note it not harshly but with curiosity. This activity of comparison may be a characteristic you learn about yourself on the mat that you can then take with you off the mat. The terms *on the mat* and *off the mat* refer to a means of reflecting on your life by using the awareness gained from your time on the yoga mat and using those insights outside of the class. Similarly, if "echolocation" is the mode you use for being okay in class, it might be the same in life. You might be assessing yourself by comparing yourself to others. We learn in the yoga studio that we can only be where we are. Of course, you want to get an idea about what "loose, comfortable clothing" is, what the poses are, how you should be situated, and how you should be breathing; however, once that is determined, the yoga instructor is your guide and your body is your teacher. Again and again you will be training yourself to come back to your own mat, and into your own body. The *yamas* and *niyamas* can help with that.

THE *YAMAS* AND *HATHA* YOGA

Hatha yoga is enhanced when incorporating the restraints (*yamas*) and the observances (*niyamas*) on the mat. Including these tools can make the physical practice of yoga rich as they also aid in one's recovery. Utilizing the *yamas* of nonharming, nonlying, nonstealing, will allow one to be in the poses in a safe way—acknowledging one's capacity. Practicing nonexcess will ensure that one stays within abilities and nonattachment will allow contentment in the poses. Incorporating these restraints allows one to focus attention on the experience of the moment, while remaining aware of the level of exertion while in each pose.

Ahimsa, nonharming, cautions us not to harm ourselves or others in thought, word, or deed, so be careful about how you address yourself in your mind, how you interpret your activity, and how you hold and express your pose. The instructions of a yoga teacher may invite you to find an idealized form and foundation in a pose. These directions are an image, the shape you are moving into. Your task is to integrate the suggestions into your pose without harming yourself. As you practice, you begin to learn the difference between the sensations of effort and the pain of harm. With the tightness and tension that exists in a recovering body, one might be tempted to push or shove past optimum limits to get into the extreme of a pose. This is ill-advised. As addicts, if we take this "more is better" attitude onto the mat, we risk injury and sacrifice growth and other benefits. In search of the extreme, we may be bringing old habits to this new arena. Observe and be aware of this. No self-reproaching. In this we also do no harm. Approach each posture gently, and it will invite you inside. Listen—and follow *ahimsa.*

Satya, or nonlying, will also guide you in how you practice yoga. Are you trying a pose without accepting a modification due to pride or stubbornness? Are you resisting guidance or encountering another one of your personal defects of character? *Satya* might ask if you are being honest with how much you exert yourself, with how far you can stretch or how long you can hold a pose. There is a delicate balance between finding the pose of nonharming and the pose of adequate or full expression; you don't want to hurt yourself, but you might need to feel the sensations of extension and effort. You might be listening to some story about yourself from the past—about your physical abilities or mental capacities. These would be outdated stories that are no longer the truth for you. Examine them, both on and off the mat. You might even tell yourself stories about your current condition: too tired or too stiff to practice, too distracted or preoccupied to give your practice full attention while on the mat. I find that these stories are often a conceit that I have created out of habit, ones that keep me from taking care of myself. Usually the untruths dissipate once I come to class, but I must be vigilant and ask myself, "Is this my full effort and attention? Can I bring my mind to this moment? May I fully engage in exploring this pose, my practice, today?"

These questions work in one's recovery program as well. There are times when you might be tempted to make excuses to avoid reading your Basic Text or recovery literature, avoid meeting with your sponsor or other recovery friends, or skip a meeting. Is this process of telling yourself stories (excuses, reasons, and justifications) similar to what you do on the mat? Are you avoiding challenging poses or holding difficult postures by telling yourself such stories? Honesty is a basic tenet in recovery as well, so practicing the nuances of this fundamental recovery principle enhances one's whole life.

Asteya, nonstealing, can take complex forms in your yoga practice. You can overreach a pose by trying to step into "tomorrow's pose"—a perfect form that will come from practice and the strength, flexibility, and breath work you cultivate today. Just as you might want the apparent ease of multiple years of recovery, you can only find that in the years to come. If you let your eyes wander around a yoga studio, you might be envious of another's pose and try, with much effort and possibly a lack of wisdom, to take it as your own. Pushing your body beyond reasonable limits is stealing from your "now" of being. At worst you could harm yourself, and at minimum you could deprive yourself of the benefits of the current state of your pose. Moving into a shape that is not your true pose may block the energy and health benefits the actual pose could provide. Forgetting the restraint of nonstealing, you might be reaching into the future, trying to take from it that which you have not already earned, which is not practicing *asteya*.

Another way you may steal from yourself is by not being fully mindful of your practice of the moment, of where you are. You might find that your body is situated on the mat, but for some reason your mind has gone on a walkabout—to the past, to the future, or to some fantasy. It may have become involved in comparing or judging—looking at other students and becoming distracted. As a less-than-flexible person, I spent the initial period of time on the mat comparing myself to the other female students, and not listening closely to my various teachers. I stole the possibility of expanding and enhancing my yoga practice due to self-centered fear and pride. Eventually I became more content with my practice just as it was on my mat, and I allowed myself to practice within my capacity. I was then opened up to the entire world of yoga practices, not just those I thought I could handle. I experienced them all, each within my own abilities, no longer letting my ego steal the opportunity from myself. This is the mental practice of *asteya*.

Finally, you might find stealing can occur when you fear scarcity. This is easier to understand off the mat, where you might take something— an object, or even somebody's idea—because you fear you can't get it any other way. On the mat this can be insidious. You might be holding back in your practice because you do not trust that you have enough strength or stamina to fully embrace a pose or continue through the set. You pull back by walking through the practice rather than resting and coming back stronger. A mindful way to address your practice could be by using the first *yama*, *ahimsa* (nonharming), to guide you: come into a child's pose, find your breath, and then return with new vigor. In this way you can be fully involved in your practice, and not stealing the full experience from yourself. Trust in the abundance of your own nature, your own strength; become balanced with *ahimsa* and *satya* to practice *asteya*.

Brahmacharya, nonexcess or nongreed, can guide wisely in our practice. Going into extremes in a pose or holding a posture so long that the breath becomes labored or ragged is excessive. One has become greedy in the pose, perhaps gauging one's own practice by comparing it to that of another person. Practicing *brahmacharya*, we utilize our internal resources without dissipating our *prana*, or energy. We equalize, or distribute, the effort by using all the muscles of the body in each pose—not just the large muscles that engage first, but all the muscles and tendons—and by using the core muscles in all we do. As we tap that inner strength and support the whole of our body, our pose can bring a calm steadiness to our practice on and off the mat. We learn to find a balance between what our body needs and what we imagine we need. As an addict I believed that "too much of a good thing was a good thing" and that "if some was good, more was better." Not only would any inebriant do, but "sufficient" quantity was not a concept that made sense. This is the crux of all addictions, the need for more—more porn, one more game of cards, one more lover, the rest of the cake, one more minute in front of the screen. Moderation is not a concept addicts understand. This is an old story that is no longer my truth, but during times when I am down and vulnerable, the old stories can sneak back into my head. Greed can manifest itself in a number of ways—not only in the physical realm, but in consumerism as well. Getting the right mat, carry bag, clothes, and accessories—all can become an obsession that focuses on the "perfect accoutrement" to bring health and recovery rather than the practice itself. This can occur in any facet of life, from cooking to crafts, bike riding to books. There are occasions when the trappings of an activity take the place of the activity itself. Watch and be aware and make good choices. So, too, I must not overdo it in my practice and overreach my capabilities, or overuse my energies beyond that which is healthy. Quietly, subtly, and with a grateful heart, greed—non-*brahmacharya*—can be avoided. The moment, the pose, and the practice can be sufficient and delicious in and of themselves.

Aparigraha, nonattachment or letting go, is an important practice in our recovery as well as in our yoga practice. It also is a tricky and subtle restraint. Beginning with the letting go of expectations—of the body, the mind, the emotions, and the spiritual effects—when practicing yoga is the first step in following this restraint. Holding on to the image of yoga models and fixed ideas about flexibility, strength, the shape of the poses in their extreme, and the shape of one's body in the present can stand in the way of a wholesome yoga practice. These types of mind stories also stand in the way of a wholesome life. How many times do we sell ourselves short or talk ourselves out of new and meaningful experiences because we are unwilling to let go of an unfounded or no-longer-relevant concept about ourselves? We continually hold on to our old ideas about our mind, body, emotions, and spirit. Let go, let go of the past, and let go of the results—and "Be Here Now," as Ram Dass says. Practicing *aparigraha,* we can stay within our own body. Being mindful of our own abilities and following the other *yamas,* we can develop a practice that is uniquely our own and acquire what we need to learn about our bodies and ourselves, each breath at a time, one day at a time, each practice at a time, with reverence.

THE *NIYAMAS* AND *HATHA* YOGA

Including the *niyamas* in *hatha* yoga enriches one's practice on a subtly personal level. Incorporating the concepts of purity, contentment, discipline, self-study, and surrender to the divine can bring a depth of mindfulness to *asana* that mere exercise cannot evince. As the *yamas* and *niyamas* interweave and reinforce each other, applying the *niyamas* deepens the yoga practice in a mindful way. The *niyamas* manifest primarily in the attitude and outlook that you take to the mat. While subtle, they can have a profound impact on your yoga practice.

Saucha, cleanliness, can include coming to the studio with an open mind, without judgment or prejudice. Stepping into the space and removing one's shoes (symbolically leaving the cares of the external world outside the practice space), being mindful of one another's mats (not stepping on them or other props), and being respectful of the studio suggestions against heavy scents or perfumes are also facets of a *saucha* practice. In order to preserve the sanctity of a practice, one might begin and end a class with a ritual such as chanting *om,* a way of sealing in the energies that are shared during a yoga class and preserving the *saucha* that has been created. Developing this sense of reverence and respect for our practice on the mat can be transferred to yourself and your relationships off the mat. Being mindful of our surroundings and those of another, as we are in the studio, and coming into communion with others while leaving behind our own issues, as we do when leaving our shoes at the door and being careful not to "step on another's toes" as we avoid stepping on another's mat, we can bring *saucha* into our recovery lives.

Santosha, contentment, is an aspiration to be enjoyed during a class. Be content in your practice. Contentment is an inside job. In the rooms of recovery, we say that self-esteem is not "other esteem"; it comes from the self. So, too, true contentment comes from within ourselves. Comparing ourselves with others, in life and on the mat, can either diminish us by our evaluating ourselves negatively when compared to another, or (falsely) make us feel better by our comparing ourselves with those we judge to be worse. This negative illusion is often a projection of our own fears. That is not contentment.

Occasionally what we like or enjoy about a teacher or a class is based on likes and dislikes of certain poses or sequences. Our attitude is what might be making the class "good" or "bad." The poses or sequences themselves are not good or bad; it is our impression or interpretation that makes them so. We find in life itself that people, places, and things might not be to our liking or choosing. It is strongly suggested that we each find a way to accept things as they are. Yoga teaches us to practice contentment and with this attitude to find peace. We may find that allowing things to be just as they are can bring contentment. Just be. In recovery we are first introduced to the concept of letting things be as they are (i.e., not becoming attached to them) in the discernment practice of "taking what you want and leaving the rest." When we go to meetings, we might find complaint, and voice it to one another. The more experienced or skilled members will smile and repeat the phrase, "Take what you want and leave the rest." Don't spend time criticizing. These members lead us to our first practice in nonjudgment. People, ideas, opinions, and words are of themselves not good or bad. We discover what is useful for us and leave what is not. When we participate in the folly of "taking another's inventory," we most often catch ourselves with knowing humor and cease without self-criticism. Most often we cease with love and understanding of our humanity. We learn to let people be as they are. We practice *santosha*.

Occasionally we find enjoyment in poses that come easily to us and avoid those that challenge us. Observe yourself; can you find contentment in accepting the challenge? While it might not be as enjoyable initially, the sense of accomplishment might bring contentment. What if you could find contentment in all the postures, allowing the feeling of effort to engage you in a positive way, just as you do the poses that flow easily out of your body? Where are you more mindful and aware? Can you cultivate those feelings of challenge and involvement and derive contentment from them—if not at the exact moment of exertion, then later during the integrative process in final relaxation, *sivasana*? Sometimes accomplishment from perseverance can give the most contentment. Though practicing the principles of the program can be daunting and challenging, we eventually find peace in the path. Observing the *niyamas* will help guide you into a space where the practice can be nurturing and fulfilling, and *santosha* can be the outcome.

Tapas, or discipline, is what moves you through the door and into right effort on the mat. Just as you can't get the program of recovery without practicing the principles and going to meetings, you can't progress in your physical yoga practice without the discipline of regular practice and a mindful level of exertion. Bring the wandering mind into the moment and into the breath by applying *tapas.* Removing all that is not essential is *tapas.* Letting go of judgment and inventory taking, of comparison and self-criticism, is also part of observing *tapas.* At times the body is the easiest thing to bring to class; the chattering mind is often out of control, preventing the whole system (body, mind, emotions, and spirit) from enjoying the benefits of the practice. The energy release and rejuvenation, which are gifts from a mindful practice, can elude one when the mind wanders or is undisciplined. Exerting energy, without the mental commentary and with focus and compassion, encourages the emotions, mind, body, and spirit to join you on the mat—in the true yoking together that is yoga.

Self-study, *svadhyaya*, is the constant companion of the practicing yogi. Remaining on your own mat, maybe even practicing with your eyes closed from time to time, enhancing inner awareness, will guide you into deeper self-study. What do you avoid and what do you crave? When do you find resistance and when do you embrace challenge? How you are on the mat is very similar to how you are in life: Do you face difficulty or avoid discomfort? Do you race headlong into things, or are you cautious and slow? Do you attempt challenging poses, or do you hold back? Are you more likely to listen to your body honestly, or do you ignore the warnings of potential injury? Knowing your proclivities and being aware of them, and when they hinder and help you, is part of the benefits of self-study that yoga brings. As you learn about your shortcomings doing the steps, you become more alert to them in life and in your dealings with people, places, and things. A mindful, steadfast study of the Twelve Steps with a sponsor or group will lead to greater knowledge about yourself and how you act in life. A steady yoga practice can open your heart, deepen your spiritual connection, and begin to release the trapped tensions in your battered body. In turn, these releases can bring a deeper understanding to your step work and self-awareness. Finding this skill on the mat and bringing it to the rest of your life is an expression of *svadhyaya*.

Surrender to the divine—*ishvara pranidhana*—is a major step in the program of recovery and a major practice in yoga. We are all divine; we are all part of the divine nature of all beings. We find our Higher Power and dedicate the outcome of our actions to that being or entity. In our *hatha* practice as well, we do our best to surrender; it is a large part of the practice. But it is important to do our best in our best way and stay out of the results. Each person will find his or her own challenge on (and off) the mat; each person will exhibit his or her own level of effort and dedication. Be mindful of exerting right effort, knowing that it will exist only in the moment, to be embraced again in the next. In final relaxation we have an opportunity to feel the effects of our practice, and in doing so we can dedicate the results of the experience to our Higher Power, grateful for our capacity to practice and unify ourselves.

A YOGA THAT SUITS YOUR RECOVERY

Various types and styles of yoga were referenced in Chapter Three and are listed in the Appendix. As with recovery meetings, not all groups appeal to all; not all formats appeal to all. When we first come into the rooms of recovery, it is suggested that we attend ninety meetings in ninety days. This not only keeps us in the rooms and away from the temptations of our addiction; we also have the opportunity to take in a lot of different meetings, meeting styles, and locations. In that process we find which types of meetings suit our style. While "ninety in ninety" is not practical for yoga classes, the same basic principle applies. Try a few different classes on a regular basis and make choices. As part of an overall plan for recovery and relapse prevention, *hatha* yoga can bring the body back to balance and reinforce the relationship among body, mind, and spirit. It may take some effort to find a yoga class or studio to which you can dedicate yourself. Taking the time to do so is invaluable.

Finding a yoga class can begin simply by asking friends. There are classes in many communities that cater specifically to people recovering from addictions. Y12SR is such a group. These classes are popping up in yoga studios and community centers all over the country. They incorporate an addiction recovery meeting with a yoga class. The first hour is a topic discussion meeting, followed by a one-hour yoga practice. There are also free-form classes that are based on bringing the *yamas* and *niyamas* into the yoga class and tying them to twelve-step recovery principles. Still other classes incorporate affirmations with the poses to promote right thinking and to change habits of the mind in more healthful and positive directions.

Don't give up on yoga: try several styles and a variety of studios until you find one that meets your needs. You may even need to try the same studio and instructor for a few classes to determine what fits you—even teachers have an off day. Allow your desire, willingness, and a positive attitude to guide you when selecting a class, just as you do when going to a new meeting. We have an expression in yoga: "Where the attention goes, the *prana* goes"—*prana* being our life-force energy. If you concentrate on the negative, it will grow and a downward spiral of negativity will ensue.

DVDs and recorded classes that you can practice with at home have some value, but the *sangha,* the community of other students and an experienced teacher, can enhance your yoga practice as meetings support your recovery. There are specific types of yoga classes, and once you get used to the language, the class descriptions can help you know what to expect. There are classes based on a flow from pose to pose: some of these are *ashtanga, vinyasa,* and *Tri Yoga.* Classes can be designed with a sequence of static poses. These may be *yin* yoga, *iyengar,* or other foundational classes. There are a variety of therapeutic yoga classes for injury recovery or prevention or for rejuvenation, such as restorative yoga, trauma release yoga (TRE), chair yoga, and Integral Therapies. There are also specific classes for

Power Yoga, Yoga Fit, and Yoga Tune Up, and there is *bikram* yoga. Let it be a journey to find out which one (or ones) suit you the best.

Finally, there is the practice of *Yoga Nidra*, which is specifically designed to relax the body and focus the mind in a progressive process of withdrawal of the senses, bringing you to a balancing point between wakefulness and sleep and allowing you to move into a state of spiritual discovery.

THE BREATH AS A TOOL

There are many documented benefits of the physical practice of yoga. According to Dr. Timothy McCall, a well-known physician who, although conventionally trained, incorporates *ayurvedic* medicine into his practice, yoga is the "one-stop shop" for health and disease prevention. The practice of *hatha* yoga increases strength, balance, flexibility, and equanimity. It also decreases stress and heart and respiration rates, and balances the nervous system. It does the same with the sympathetic nervous system—the "fight-or-flight" response—and the parasympathetic nervous system, which relaxes you, allowing you to become balanced with the mindful combination of pose sequences and control of the breath. The breath practices— breathing in and out through the nose (breathing through the mouth is only done for specialized breath work)—warm, humidify, and filter the breath. Yoga brings consciousness to the mind and body connection in a process known as "somatics." Experiences and tensions that were locked in the muscles and joints are released with consistent movement and mindful attention to the body. This can bring physical and emotional relief. There are times in a yoga practice when emotions erupt. One may feel sad or angry, or experience some other intense emotion. Having the courage to stay with the feelings is important; you are not a freak or alone in having this kind of experience. It may not even matter *why* the feelings are coming out—it is a grace that they do emerge. Once the feelings, the sensations, are processed, the body can move more freely; the breath can move more easily and completely. Energy levels may improve after the release of previously blocked emotions, and a new level of enjoyment may emerge. Removing the obstructions to the flow of energy through the body allows for smoother, deeper breathing.

Breathing in a full and efficient manner calms the brain and enhances neurological activity. An agitated mind is not an efficient mind. Increasing the effectiveness of the breathing process expands mental acuity. Moving the joints and stimulating the glands in the body also promote health. Rotating each major joint, testing and increasing range of motion, building strength in the muscles, and moving the spine judiciously on a daily basis will heal and rejuvenate the body. Twists and compression/release of the abdominals can detoxify the body and promote healthy digestion. After a lifetime of abusing the body with substances or in blatant disregard for its health and needs, practicing these poses and movements can help return the body to good physical condition.

The most important part of yoga is regular practice. As with recovery and consistent attendance at meetings, progress is found only with a consistent attention. As you may have discovered after steady meeting attendance, you find you *need* to attend meetings; there is a total sense of longing when too much time has passed between meetings. Likewise, your body and internal serenity may urge you, through a similar longing, to join in a yoga practice. Your body may feel tight or congested, and this discomfort may beckon you back to the mat. The quietness of mind found in this beneficial practice may also lure you back to yoga. Loosening and invigorating the body, learning deeper and more efficient ways to breathe, and finding the pure relaxation in the final pose—*savasana*—will lead you easily into that elusive practice: meditation.

EXERCISE

ASANA

In *asana* practice you can begin by taking a moment to set an intention: a wish or prayer for yourself. This is conventionally a long-term goal or aspiration such as developing patience, self-acceptance, compassion, or gratitude. Find something that suits you and incorporate that into your breath and movement.

In warming up before your practice, take quadruped—hands and knees pose—then inhale into cow pose and exhale into cat pose three to five times, moving slowly between the two. Come to standing. Finding standing mountain pose, *tadasana*, begin a mindful review of the posture from the equilibrium of your feet on the earth through the strength of the legs, the engagement of the core, the softness of the shoulders and collarbones, to the balance of your head on the top of your spine. Be aware of the integrity of your physical body and mind. On an inhale, raise your arms in upward salute, soften the knees, and exhale into a forward fold. Repeat several times, straightening the legs in the final round if your hamstrings will allow it. Proceed to performing a few swings at the waist, rotating from side to side, keeping the legs and pelvis stationary and allowing the arms and shoulders to swing freely. Repeat these movements ten to twenty times from side to side. Prepare your mind and body to move into static poses.

There are four parts to every yoga pose: coming into the pose, being in the pose, coming out of the pose, and being in between the poses. Repeat each of the poses below several times, each time bringing to mind a different *yama* or a *niyama*. Use the ones suggested or select ones of your own. Coming into *tadasana* between each repetition, use the pause between the poses to reiterate the concept and bring it home, recalling a situation or challenge in your own life.

1. Stepping the right foot back, come into pyramid pose (*parsvotton asana*). Contemplate *ahimsa* (nonharming), and *saucha* (cleanliness). Keep precision in your pose and come to each awareness with a clean intention—an intention of self-growth and health rather than the extreme of the physical pursuit. The challenge of this forward fold can remind you to do your best but to refrain from doing too much. Repeat on the left side. Alternate between the two sides a few more times.

2. Stepping the right foot back, adjust the stance to prepare for crescent pose (high lunge, or modified with right knee to the ground). Bending the left knee so that it comes over the left ankle, raise the arms above the head. The heart is open in crescent; mindfulness and compassion can enter and support you in this pose of strength and expansion. Calling on *satya*—truthfulness—find the depth and length of the pose that is honestly yours. Do not aspire to go too deep or be too moderate. Bring *ahimsa* into each and every pose; bring honesty into your effort. *Santosha*, or contentment, advises that we find peace with where we are. If the mind drifts off the mat to images or remembrances of other people, other times, and other poses, beckon it to your mat and the present moment. The balance between honesty and contentment is the balance of effort and ease sought in a physical practice,

in our emotional health, and in our spiritual condition. Use the silence and the pause in between the repetitions to find the applications of these tenets in your life and your recovery. Repeat with left leg stepping back. Repeat again a few times on each side.

3. Step the right foot back and set the feet into proper position for triangle pose (*utthita trikonasana*). Breathe into *asteya,* nonstealing, again exerting right effort, and with that use *tapas,* or discipline, ensuring that you bring the transformational intention to the pose. Triangle is a powerful brain-balancing pose. It combines the downward strength and power of the legs with elongation of the spine, opening of the heart, and expansion of the arms and chest. As you breathe into today's expression of the pose and hold the pose as long as the breath remains fluid and smooth, think about the concepts and apply them physically. When you return to *tadasana,* contemplate the tenets as they apply to your recovery and your spiritual journey. Do the pose on the left side, then repeat a few times on each side.

4. From standing mountain, step the right foot back and come into extreme side-angle pose (*utthita parsvakonasana*). The name of this pose might lead you to believe that you must practice to the extreme. That is not true: while the line of the pose is extreme, the effort should be just right. Practice *brahmacharya,* nonexcess, in this demanding pose. There are a score of minor physical adjustments that can be made when opening into this pose. Bringing all other *yamas* and *niyamas* to mind, move into this pose and hold it with respect for yourself, your effort, and your serenity. Examine how you are in this pose—let this be an opportunity for *svadhyaya,* the skill of self-study. As you remain in the pose, be aware of

the desire either to come out of the pose or to overcome or conquer the pose. Does this give you information about how you approach life? Return to *tadasana*, reflect, and move to the other side. Repeat each side a few times. Pause and contemplate how your body feels and note where your mind has gone. Do this with curiosity, searching for information, and without judgment.

5. Come onto all fours into quadruped. Tucking the toes, come up into downward-facing dog (*adho mukha svanasana*). Lengthen the back and invite the heels toward the mat. Let the head hang without effort. Breathe smoothly and embrace the integration that this pose offers. Over time, downward-facing dog will become a posture of rest and reinvigoration. Initially there is a lot of effort involved in remaining centered. Take this time to let go—the principle of *aparigraha*. Let the neck and head hang and allow the strength from the four attachments to the mat ground you. Equalize the exertion between hands and feet, right side and left side. Do your best and let go of the results. Allow the pose to "grow on you" in *ishvara pranidhana:* surrender. When you are ready to come out of the pose, come back to quadruped. Repeat several times, coming back to all fours and remaining there in between. Take these moments in between the effort-sustained pose to see how you can integrate the ideas of letting go and surrender in your life. When moving into the pose, see where these concepts move into your body.

Back and forth: mind, spirit, and body.

From quadruped, stretch out on the mat on your belly. Bring the hands next to your chest, fingertips under your shoulder. Legs extended on the mat, lower back drawing away from the shoulders, use the muscles of the back to rise into cobra/

salabhasana. Use the strength of the back to rise up. Gaze is down or slightly forward; keep the back of the neck smooth for this variation of cobra. Remain here for three breaths, then lie down, bringing the bent arms forward, stacking the hands and putting one cheek on the hands for a full round of breath to rest. Repeat this pose three more times, alternating which cheek is on the stacked hands for the resting part of the sequence. Return to all fours.

6. To conclude your practice:

From all fours, reach your hips back to your heels, come into child's pose, and rest for a moment. Roll onto your right hip, swing your legs out in front of you, and sit with a tall spine. Coming onto your back by using the arms for support, lie down and draw your knees to your chest. Rock side to side a few times before coming into simple twist for several breaths on each side. From back-lying pose, extend each leg onto the floor, make yourself comfortable, and come into corpse pose, *savasana*, for a minimum of five minutes. Allow yourself to relax completely, come out slowly, and respect your newfound state.

CHAPTER EIGHT

Pranayama

PRANAYAMA: BREATH PRACTICES AND CONTROL (OR MANAGEMENT)

Patanjali tells us, "The breath transcends the level of the consciousness," and that the "regular practice of *pranayama* reduces the obstacles that inhibit clear perception" (2.51 and 2.52). Correct and conscious breathing clarifies the mind.

There are lots of benefits from *pranayama*, so how do we find effective breathing? We have been breathing all our life long, which goes without saying, but how have we been breathing? Understanding more about respiration may help in our investigation and encourage us to adopt better breathing practices.

A root word of *pranayama, prana,* is not just breath, but the energy that the breath creates. The depth, pace, and rhythm of the breath influence how the energy is utilized and distributed through the body. They influence how the oxygen is utilized by the brain. It is important to address the HOW of our breathing, its depth and duration, our natural rhythm. In general, particularly in the Western cultures where we have not given much attention to breath control, we breathe in a shallow manner, either high in the chest or into the belly without involving the rib area. Either way of breathing allows only a small amount of oxygen into our lungs with each inhale. In addition, we may be breathing in a fairly rapid or uneven manner, preventing the body from absorbing all it can from each breath. If you bring your attention to your breath right now, you will notice a subtle change—an increase in the depth and the duration of each cycle—merely as the result of bringing your consciousness to your breath. You intuitively know the more beneficial way to breathe; it is the habit of our culture, our lifestyle, or our mind that prevents us from breathing fully.

BREATH MECHANICS

There is a direct connection between breathing (lung function) and cell development/regeneration and our neurological responses to situations. There are a few complex activities happening simultaneously. The oxygen in the blood is absorbed through the lungs. Bringing an adequate amount of breath into the lungs and allowing it to remain there for a sufficient period of time for the exchange to occur is necessary for the optimum transmission of oxygen. The efficiency of this whole process has an impact on the physical body, starting with the response and strength of muscles. Further, the breath greatly affects the nervous system, which is divided into the somatic and the autonomic nervous systems. It is the latter that we focus on when we discuss breath and breathing patterns. The autonomic nervous system is divided into two branches, the parasympathetic and the sympathetic nervous systems. The former controls the resting activities, such as digestion, and it calms, slows, and quiets the functions of the body. The sympathetic nervous system governs the active, externally directed functions, such as our response to an emergency situation or physical exercise. It energizes, contracts, and moves us. These systems do not function simultaneously, as our energies and actions move in a cycle between the two, alternating between energizing and relaxing the body. If we experience trauma, we can become stuck in one of the modes: either retreating into a "freeze" or parasympathetic condition, or striking out in the fight-or-flight syndrome of the sympathetic nervous system. The body needs to experience either a parasympathetic or a sympathetic discharge, and then cycle back to the other. An interruption of this cyclical process causes the *prana*, or energy, to be trapped in the body. We can experience negative physical and neurological results from these blockages. (See such works as *Healing Trauma*, by Peter Levine, *The Revolutionary Trauma Release Process* by David Berceli, or *Unlocking Your Body* by Thomas Hanna among others who have written on somatic psychology and somatic therapy.)

So what happens to our body, our mind, and our emotions with short, shallow breaths? We are stuck in the fight-or-flight mode: a state of constant agitation, alertness, and anxiety. We are looking for something to happen. Early in recovery we may feel that we are constantly waiting for the other shoe to drop, never feeling settled, constantly ready for something else to happen. If your drugs of choice were "uppers," like amphetamines or cocaine, this state of agitation may have become a new normal. If gambling or any other risky behavior was your addiction, again, feelings of being hyper-alert and energized are quite familiar. In fact, those feelings may have become a form of craving. You have learned to yearn for those feelings or for being anxious, rushed, or overcommitted, as these feelings have become the "new normal." Shallow breathing also contributes to an inability to properly think though situations. The stimulation of the sympathetic nervous system is designed for quick reactions, with little or no time for thought or consideration. Habitual actions dominate. For those of us who got stuck in the "on" position, decisions were faulty, reactions were excessive, and the body got worn out—all the energies and *prana* were depleted through this continual abuse.

For those who get stuck in the "freeze" position, shallow breathing has depleted *prana*. Being unfocused and fearful, sluggish, and lethargic are ways this imbalance can be manifested. If your addictive behavior included isolating activities like video gaming, or if your drugs of choice were "downers" like heroin or prescription medication, you may feel withdrawn and have difficulty engaging with others. Your body may be lethargic and lacking in energy. You may have difficulty making decisions, and this can have dangers of its own, especially in emergency situations. Shallow breathing can deprive the brain of valuable oxygen, perpetuating this soporific condition and contributing to an inability to respond quickly to situations.

WHAT THE BREATH CAN DO

Learning how to breathe, to breathe deeply with various techniques that involve and invigorate the body and the brain, can be life-changing. I have had numerous yoga students comment to me on the enormous positive impact that breath practice has had on them. "I wanted to let you know I breathed all week long," said one student. Another commented, "I was feeling angry and I remembered what you said about breathing; I took a few breaths and realized it was no big deal," and "It made me feel more clear-minded."

I am the sort of person who rushes headlong into things. I rush into activities, conversations, opinions, and life. As I moved into recovery, I had to learn to pause, to take stock, to inhale and exhale and "test the air around me," and to assess a situation before I reacted. I needed to learn how to sit with my feelings, reactions, and the occasional discomfort. I did this by learning to breathe through the unknown and sit in the present moment and mind state. *Pranayama,* conscious breath control, taught me that skill. Many of us may have heard from our mothers or grandmothers, "Take ten breaths before you act." What good advice. Just taking time to breathe can give you a moment to reflect—on the situation and on your own response. It can give you time to consciously choose. Breath soothes the mind and calms the body. Mindful breathing can allow one to withdraw from the immediacy of the moment, to respond rather than react.

The qualities of each breath cycle are for it to be smooth and even, deep and slow, quiet, and without any jerks or pauses. This is achieved first by listening. Ganga White states in his book *Yoga Beyond Belief* that "breathing is both conscious and unconscious. . . . We cannot even think about the breath without influencing it and without it coming back under conscious control."[1] Listen to your breath, note that it is now under your control, and begin to investigate your breathing patterns. The next step is to consciously influence your breathing with some specific patterns designed to enhance your breathing apparatus and other methods designed to affect emotions and energies. There are breath practices created to invigorate you, and others that calm and relax you. Some breath controls support your *asana* practice, others your meditations. White goes on to suggest that you be aware of your breath in *asana* and discern what difference the breath can make in your poses. Some breath work can have transcendent properties, like alternating-nostril breathing, when practiced over a period of time under the guidance of a skilled teacher. And there are breathing techniques that can help you work long and at a steady pace. Breath work is used in pain management as well in the treatment of anxiety disorders. It requires practice and patience. It is a powerful tool to add to your repertoire.

There are breath control practices that can exaggerate any of the four parts of breathing—the inhalation (*paruka* in Sanskrit), the pause after inhaling (*abhyantara kumbhaka*), the exhalation (*rechaka*), or the pause after exhale (*bahya kumbhaka*).

ENGLISH DESCRIPTION OF BREATH	SANSKRIT TERM
Inhalation	*Pukara*
Pause at the top of the inhale	*Antara kumbhaka*
Exhalation	*Rechaka*
Pause with the breath outside the body	*Bahya kumbhaka*

There are practices that combine control of each one of these four facets with blockage of the nostrils, glottis, or diaphragm, or manipulation of the tongue. While some breathing techniques are described here, it is very useful to have an experienced teacher help with their practice. As mentioned earlier, the effect of the breath in the body is that it releases energy. It is helpful to have someone who can help you understand the feelings that arise and the effects when you experience these releases. While these can include enhancement of well-being and peace of mind, reduction in levels of stress, support of the immune system, increased optimism, relief of anxiety and depression (mild, moderate, and severe), enhanced brain function (increased mental focus, calmness), and increased speed of recovery from stressful stimuli, there can also be emotional releases from past traumas that require care and understanding to process.

BREATHING TECHNIQUES

There are several classic yoga breathing systems. Victorious breath (*ujjai*), three-part "yoga" breath (*dhirgha*), alternating-nostril breathing (*nadi shodhana*), shining face or shining skull breath (*kapalabhati*), bellows breathing (*bhakstrika*), and buzzing-bee breath (*bhramari*) are some of the various breath control methods. Most breathing techniques take years of practice for them to achieve maximum effectiveness. The uses are specific to certain aims, such as heating the body, calming the mind, aiding digestion, promoting circulation in the internal organs, or cooling the body and the mind. Some of the breath practices have been described in the Exercise section of previous chapters; still others should be learned face-to-face with an experienced practitioner to ensure that the complexities of the practice are understood. There are certain breath practices that involve a suction or "lock," preserving the energy within the body. An exhale with a suction that pulls the belly in and up behind the ribs is such a practice used in *uddiyana bandha*. It takes some comfort and ease with other breath practices before moving into these more complex breathing styles.

One gains skill in the less complex breath control practices in order to explore the more difficult ones. In my old way of thinking as an addict, I would have imagined that I could both

1. learn them myself without the aid of a teacher; and

2. do them more robustly and with greater frequency than prescribed.

This is an unhelpful and unhealthy way of thinking—using the old "more is better" ideation. I caution you to defer to better judgment and find a skilled practitioner in order that the breath practice bring you its genuine benefits and that you do not do harm to yourself.

USING THE *YAMAS* AND *NIYAMAS* IN YOUR BREATH PRACTICE

Approach your practice of a breathing technique with the *yamas* in mind. Include the restraints of nonharming—be certain you learn the technique correctly. Be truthful and practice it to the best of your ability. Do not steal the experience from yourself: use the breath practice in a mindful way in the proper circumstance—the energizing breaths when appropriate and the soothing breaths when they are needed. Do not overuse a breath practice. Moderation is the key. While there are discernable psychic benefits from the breath practices, do not overdo it, looking for that "high feeling." Let go of any expectation for a breath practice. Like *asana* practice, the benefits make themselves known over time. Be patient and watch the magic unfold.

Bring also the mindfulness of the *niyamas* into your *pranayama.* Some techniques are specifically for cleansing purposes: *kapalibata,* or "shining face," for example. Perform this practice for the purpose intended, and you will reap the benefits. Utilize the proper breathing practices when you are doing *asana;* allow the breath to support you. While engaged in your *asana,* mindfully employing the breath, experience the contentment that proper breathing can bring. Find that sweet balance between effort and ease. Practice a specific *pranayama* for a period of time with dedication, bringing *tapas* to your work. Be mindful and curious about what occurs when you do use your breath practice regularly and when you don't. Investigate why you don't adhere to your practice schedule when you choose to forgo this beautiful part of your yoga. Without judgment, learn from this, practicing the *niyama* of *svadhyaya.* Finally comes *ishvara pranidhana,* surrender: give yourself over to the practice and give the result to your Higher Power, always doing the best you can and letting go of the outcome. In this way you can bring the *niyamas* to your *pranayama.*

Bringing breath awareness to your life can also alert you to your true feelings—help you to discern the source of unpleasant feelings when you have them. Discover if what you are really experiencing is hunger, anger, loneliness, or just being tired. Are you breathless, is your chest tight, are you anxious and forgetting to bring the full breath into your body and allowing it to linger there before the exhale? We can revert to old habits when we are under stress, allowing old ways of thinking to invade our best intentions. Compounding this old-timey thinking with old breathing habits can upset the chemical balance in the mind, making it feel like the old way. Deprived of oxygen, your chemistry moves into the fight-or-flight mode, upsetting right thinking and right action. Use this new awareness as a tool. The yoga of *pranayama* can bring you to the mindfulness of HALT. When feelings mount up, when reactions are becoming increasingly overblown, when what you want for your new, recovered self is being sabotaged by your "old" self, breathe.

• Are you in fact "running on empty"?

• Have you used up your emotional or energetic reserves?

• Have you allowed a situation to exceed your capacity to respond to and cope with it, with the result that you have become ready to coil and spring?

• Would a break, a time for tea and reflection or a meal and a moment, or even a nap be possible?

• Can you take ten breaths before you give a response?

When practicing the Tenth Step to evaluate my day, I have never looked back and wished I had used harsh words when I had not. I have never looked back wishing I had been punishing or humorously vicious when I had the chance. I have, however, reflected on a situation and wished I had *not* used certain words, phrases, expressions, or humorous derision in a response. A few breaths would have saved me from a situation that may, indeed, now require an amend. As we advise in the rooms of recovery, we should practice "restraint of tongue and pen." I have heard this caution expanded on at meetings to include hitting "send" in an email. There are many ways and modalities in which we can snap back at people, where a long breath could have prevented an abrupt reaction from occurring. Taking care with my breath and being mindful of my breathing bring me home to myself, to a space where I can find my honest self, the true kernel of my being—that part of me that does not change from situation to situation or from time to time. Practicing *pranayama* for a period of time now, I can be calm and listen, and "do the next right thing."

EXERCISE

TWO-TO-ONE BREATH REGULATION

Select a time of day to devote to your breath practice: first thing in the morning or last thing at night are both good times. Sitting tall on the floor or on a straight-back chair, take a few moments to become situated with erect carriage, feet flat on the floor and head balanced on the neck, chin tucked and back of neck long. The crown of the head should reach upward.

Breathing in and out through the nose, begin by becoming aware of the breath. Invite it to become deeper, slower, and fuller with each inhale. Without stress or strain, continue in this manner for about ten breaths, just breathing and being aware of the breath.

Now begin to count slowly to yourself on the inhale, hold for one count, exhale, and hold the breath outside the body for one count.

Continue this counting for three cycles. On the fourth cycle, adjust the exhale to be of equal count to the inhale: if your count for inhale is three, hold for the count of one, exhale to the count of three, and hold outside the body for one count. Do this three times.

After the fourth inhale and one-count hold, extend the exhale by one extra count. Your new pattern may look like this: three, one, four, one. Continue like this for three to five rounds.

The next change will be to increase the exhale by another count so that the new pattern becomes three, one, five, one. After three to five rounds, increase again by one count on the exhale: three, one, six, one. Maintain this pattern for ten rounds or more.

You then decrease the exhale by one count every three to five rounds until the inhale and exhale are equal. Return to your native breath depth and duration for several rounds to complete.

NOTE: If your inhale count is another number—say, four or five—then you continue the increase until the exhale is double: eight or ten. In this manner your breath capacity increases over time and the duration of the inhale/exhale cycle can increase.

CHAPTER EIGHT NOTES

[1] White, Ganga. *Yoga Beyond Belief: Insights to Awaken and Deepen Your Practice.* Berkeley, CA: North Atlantic Books, 2007, p. 101.

CHAPTER NINE

Pratyahara, Dharana, Dhyana, and Samadhi

PRATYAHARA, DHARANA, DHYANA, AND SAMADHI TRANSLATE to withdrawal of the senses, contemplation, meditation, and bliss.

The last four limbs on the path of *raja* yoga are interdependent and intertwined with one another just as the previous limbs are, and, like those four, they cannot be practiced in isolation: each leads to and through the other. They also bring in skills acquired in the first four limbs and weave them all together. *Pratyahara, dharana,* and *dhyana,* along with the practices of the *yamas, niyamas, asana,* and *pranayama,* can lead to a blissful state. This bliss, *samadhi,* is itself the fulfillment of the promise of yoga: union of body, mind, and spirit merged with the universe. As the "promises" of Alcoholics Anonymous are fulfilled "if we work for them," so too, the gifts of yoga will be ours with practice. Mark Stephens writes in his book *Teaching Yoga*,[1] "Various strands of yoga philosophy offer different maps to attaining *samadhi*; most offer a path through *pratyahara*, *dharana*, and *dhyana* . . . useful tools for helping students cultivate clearer self-awareness, self-understanding, and self-acceptance, which, taken together, tend to yield a steadier, easier, and ultimately happier and more meaningful life." The benefits of *samadhi* are the benefits of a life in recovery from our addiction: a happier and more meaningful life.

The investigation of this path begins with understanding the differences among withdrawal of the senses, concentration, and meditation. The ultimate discovery of bliss and union will come with and through these practices.

PRATYAHARA: WITHDRAWAL OF THE SENSES

Pratyahara is a practice of withdrawing from all that is outside and all that is inside. The initial step is to pull away from stimulation of the senses, to hear and then not to hear the sounds from outside, to see and then to ignore the sense of sight, and so on. This is a process that leads from a practiced attention to inattention. Many of us have had the experience of living on a busy street. A friend may come to visit and say to us, "How can you live with all the noise? Doesn't the traffic bother you?" And you reply, "The traffic? Oh, I don't really hear it anymore." You listened to it at one time and then you didn't. Or you may work in a garden center in which there is a strong smell of fertilizer. You may be asked how you can stand the smell—and again, you may answer that you really cannot smell it anymore. These are times when your repeated exposure dulled your perception. Later you may come to use this skill consciously. In a yoga class, during final relaxation, you may be invited to listen to the sounds around you and then to let them go. You begin to withdraw the senses into your interior landscape using conscious thought. Your attention to the world around you drops away.

With my addiction to substances and also to people and relationships, I have had various experiences with the practice of *pratyahara.* In one circumstance, with the abuse of drugs and alcohol, I practiced my own diseased version of *pratyahara.* I looked for all the ways I could find to remove myself from conscious thinking and feeling, from conscious attention to my surroundings and the needs of my family and my friends. I used artificial substances in my perverted application of "withdrawal of the senses." I became sense-less. The diseased manner of withdrawal of the senses dulled and damaged my true self. On the other hand, in my codependent relationships, first with my parents, later in love, and finally with my children, I was overly attached to inputs from others. I needed their approval. I had little distinction between their feelings and needs and my own. I had to learn true *pratyahara:* to withdraw from the slightest change in facial expression, the tread of a foot, the sound of a sigh—all of which had given me cues as to how I should feel and act. I was super-tuned in to other people and took their expressions as a mandate to be involved. I was to cure, salve, solve, and control the actions and feelings of those around me. This was whether they wanted it or not. I was enmeshed. *Pratyahara* gave me the ability to let go and recover from my codependence with others and myself. The yogic withdrawal of the senses was a start to practicing healthier relationships.

Pratyahara also teaches us to avoid the overstimulation of sight, sound, touch, smell, and taste—our attachment to them and their distraction—in preparation for unfettered concentration and undisturbed meditation. On the recovery path, I needed to learn both how to hold on to necessary information I receive from the senses and also to let go of my reliance on this stimulation. On the one hand, I was very skilled at pursuing the desired effects of *pratyahara* (withdrawal through substance abuse); yet on the other, I had no boundaries and was very unskilled in relating to others, searching constantly for cues from them. The practice of *pratyahara* helped bring me back into balance, finding that place where I let go of outside stimulation as both a call to action and an escape.

Pratyahara does not require compete stillness, and it can be part of what we do when we home in and focus on one thing and all else fades away. This practice occurs when we are on the mat. We are in a difficult pose; we bring the attention to our breath and the discomfort fades away. It can happen when we are meditating—such as when we don't realize that our foot has gone to sleep—having withdrawn from any sense of the physical body. The healthy practice of *pratyahara*, moving inward away from the senses of hearing, feeling, taste, touch, and seeing, must be practiced. With steady attention, one day it will occur without force. It will meet you where you are. While I cannot force my withdrawal from and a ceasing of craving for alcohol, I can practice the conditions that will allow this sense of craving to leave me.

The power of thoughts and intentions to set our course is great. While I cannot "think myself into right action" (although I can "act myself into right thinking"), I must be aware of the power of my thoughts. Thinking can create an emotional reaction; I can scare myself and lead myself into rationalizations, i.e., talk myself out of and into things. My mind is a powerful tool. We know the power of thought in twelve-step programs of addiction recovery. We are cautioned not only to physically "stay away from slippery places," but to avoid "stinkin' thinkin'." These, too, are forms of *pratyahara*. It is important to have the ability to withdraw. Pulling away from unhealthy thinking is a step that can move us into a position to move inside, deeply, in a healthy way.

There are specific practices that may allow us to practice withdrawal of the senses. We can sit in silence, allowing the senses to drop away—touch, sight, smell, and hearing. We can also practice a more extended form of *pratyahara* by participating in a thirty- to ninety-minute-long guided form of yoga called *Yoga Nidra*. A practitioner will take the student through a series of body awareness, mind awareness, and visualization exercises to bring about total *pratyahara*. This practice can induce deep relaxation and is most achievable and enjoyable when done with a leader. In the last year of my active addiction, as I was trying desperately to "fix" my drinking and using—not to give it up but to bring it under control—I went to a therapist. In my state of economic disrepair, I went to a free clinic staffed by loving interns. There I was referred to someone who was working on her degree and who used a type of *Yoga Nidra* to relax and soothe her clients. For twenty minutes she talked me through a series of steps to identify sights, sounds, and other senses and then to let them drop away. She ushered me into deep relaxation through my breath in this process. I had not relaxed in years. I was in bliss. I did not fall asleep but fell into ease, into a bright awareness of the present moment and of her voice, letting go of everything. I was focused, awake, and relaxed. I have never forgotten the vividness of that experience. She moved on to other clinics and I didn't see her again, and I got back into my disease and did not experience that gift again until I started practicing yoga.

Pratyahara is a vital step up to the next two limbs on the *raja* path—*dharana* and *dhyana*. *Dharana* is concentration and *dhyana* is meditation. All three limbs are the process of moving inward—the most discerning and demanding of the yoga practices.

DHARANA: CONCENTRATION

Dharana is an often-overlooked and incredibly important practice: concentration. On the mat we bring the focus of our concentration to the poses. We can become acutely aware of their foundation, our effort, our ease, and the breath. This is total concentration. It is mind-body awareness at its most acute. *Pratyahara* is the starting point of this practice as you let go of everything that is not relevant to the single-pointed purpose at the moment. The mind is a busy, busy place. Thoughts fly through the mind seemingly at a million miles an hour—we actually process hundreds of thoughts a minute. Being able to concentrate on one thing at a time is a skill that improves with practice and diminishes with disuse.

You have had the experience of "being at one with the moment," being entirely in union with what you were doing—cooking, walking, creating, reading, listening to music—where you had near-complete concentration on a single thing. When the concentration on that thing or that activity is pure, then a state of *dharana* has been achieved. If there is a process of analysis—comparison, discernment, remembering the past, and forecasting into the future—then the concentration has been broken, and the seduction of the future or the past, or what things could be or are not, has taken the attention away from what IS. This bringing of the attention to a single point is both a conscious and unconscious activity. We unconsciously find single-pointed concentration in what we are doing, through the dropping away from everything else around us. We can do this in the garden when we are totally in the garden—not in other gardens or wishing our garden were something other than it is, weedless or with other blooms—but just when we forget we are there and yet remain there. We practice it when we are doing *asana*, feeling inside our bodies and reflecting on the poses as we integrate them into our still bodies. We lose this in our *hatha* practice when we look around with judging or comparing eyes. We practice this concentration when we quietly listen to the words of others at meetings—listening to them without attachment to their process or their pain—just letting them be and being purely in that moment.

There are yoga techniques one can use to increase the ability to concentrate. Some of these are *trataka*, *drishti*, and *mantra*.

1. *Trataka*—Candle flame concentration. Sit in a comfortable upright position and place a candle at eye level on a table in front of you. Gaze upon a candle flame with unblinking eyes for thirty to sixty seconds (length of time will increase with practice). When the eyes begin to experience discomfort or to water, close them and imagine the flame in your mind for thirty to sixty seconds. Open your eyes and continue, back and forth, three to six times, lengthening the duration of the opened eyes and the length of the practice over time.

2. *Drishti*—Gaze practice. Sit in a comfortable upright position. Cast the eyes down to the tip of your nose and allow the focus to soften. Hold this concentration until you feel tension building up between the eyes. Close the eyes and visualize the tip of your nose for ten to fifteen seconds, then open your eyes and resume the soft gaze. Repeat this several times.

3. *Mantra*—Finding a sound or a succession of notes to listen to or to repeat silently to ourselves is another tool for the mind to increase focus and to decrease the number of senses that are being engaged.

These methods are useful for withdrawing the mind from the outside interruptions, finding only one sense to stimulate and focusing the mind consciously on that sense.

DHYANA: MEDITATION

Meditation is not well understood. It is amazingly simple and extremely difficult. The steps of *pratyahara* (letting go of the senses and turning inward) and *dharana* (concentration) are preludes to going into meditation. There are several good books on the subject; there are CDs, DVDs, websites, and groups all devoted to enhancing one's ability to meditate. So what is meditation? It is more than concentration on the breath, a sound, a phrase or mantra, or a motif/ visual element. Meditation occurs with the noting and acceptance of the mind and body just as they are rather than indulging the addict's habit of controlling an experience. Just witnessing the present moment is an important part of meditation. Meditation occurs the moment after concentration when the candle flame, soft gaze, sound, or object in our mind leaves us. It is objectless, formless, and content consciousness–free. It includes the practice of acknowledging the thoughts and letting them go. There is a subchapter in Ganga White's book *Yoga Beyond Belief* titled "(There Is No) How to Meditate."[2] This title captures the idea of perfections and restrictions beautifully.

I struggled with the idea of the "perfect meditation practice" for years. I wanted to be an Eleventh Step "pro." I had incorporated the idea of setting an intention with the concept of "open-ended" prayer for Step Eleven, but I was struggling with the meditation part. It was mysterious. People talked about it at meetings but never with the clear specifics of *how* they did it. I read about meditation; I took a class, but sitting alone in my house, I would find my mind wandering and, squirming with physical discomfort, I'd give up after only a few minutes time and time again. It took dedicated yoga practice for me to be patient with the process: the letting go, the focus, and then the acceptance of my mental workings, such as they were, to come to a place of comfort and ease. Then I could begin to reap the benefits. I wasn't perfect; there was no perfect way and that was . . . perfect in itself.

In those moments of integration when meditation is embraced, it can lead us to the pure white light of our interior that exists within and beyond our self. There is only observation, with no attachments or judgments. This is a very important part of meditation: letting go of the judging mind. Witnessing the thoughts, acknowledging their existence, and then releasing them is the practice. Your personal distractions, the seduction of the future, the replaying of the past, being in a place of fantasy, and even repetitive self-recrimination are all mental activities that prevent us from being in the meditative state.

Addicts are seekers. Many addicts had started a meditation practice while still under the influence. This may not have brought the benefits of meditation that one can find in recovery. A besotted mind is not a clear mind, and while there can be some psychic relief from the symptoms of suffering, the true benefits of oneness and integration with all beings are not likely to occur when we are polluted by toxins or self-destructive behavior. Other people have retreated into meditation practice as a form of either relief or escape from life. This, too, has limited benefits, as attachment and aversion are forms of illusion that cloud the mind and prevent that clear, one-pointed focus that brings one from the conscious practice to the unconscious union. Even in recovery, I had to examine both my need for the "perfect practice" and my inclination toward the "more is better" school of thought. A long period of meditation practiced frequently throughout the day is a wonderful practice at a retreat, but in my current life and lifestyle, it can be a form of escape. Even with meditation, I needed to practice moderation.

While providing relief from stress and negative thinking, meditation has benefits beyond stress relief. Part of the practice of meditation comes from looking at the mind and seeing its qualities and habits. Observing the mind allows you to see what it is doing in order to accept it and let it go. While you meditate you can detect certain ways your mind gets attracted away from the breath or ways the mind moves and becomes disturbing. Here are some patterns you might find (based on the work of Swami Sitaramananda):

- *The thoughts may be unclear.* While practicing an addictive behavior or taking a substance, the mind is unlikely to be clear. Dropping the illusions that addictions create will allow the mind the possibility of clearing. The murkiness may be removed.

- *There is a phrase, "The mind is like a drunken monkey."* It jumps around from one thought to the next with wild abandon. When I am thinking about scoring dope, having sex, holding a winning poker hand, or even planning a meal or folding laundry, my mind is off on its own, mentally pursuing some sensual distraction.

- *The mind gallops off in its own direction, following thought trails one after the other.* It avoids any type of control or restriction. In recovery we all know how wrong thinking can result from a runaway mind, leading us down dark thought alleys. We learn to gently pull it back to wellness. We do not overreact by denying we have a galloping mind, thereby creating more negative energy; we just kindly call it back.

- *Sometimes the mind is shy and retiring. It still has an impact on our feelings and emotions, yet the specifics of the thoughts remain obscure.* There are parts of our true selves that have been pushed to the back of the mind, obscured by untruths and stories from our drinking, using, and other unhealthy behaviors. Our true self can also be shielded as a defense against past traumas. Be gentle. Sit quietly and let this part of yourself be known and accept it. We must know who we are in the present moment before we can choose to change.

• *The mind can fall into repetitive grooves, entertaining the same thing over and over again.* The *samskara*, or ruts, of the mind become deeper and deeper each time we go over them. In recovery the thoughts may circle around and around the record: from memories about the past to self-recrimination, to fear, and possibly to resentments, and then to guilt, around and around again. We need to find the current truth, the new thought patterns, the wiser ways of thinking, and create new, positive grooves.

• *Sometimes the mind spins; one thought flashes by, leaving a trail of feeling, and is immediately replaced by another thought.* Whisking by faster than you could imagine, possible ideas, situations, and remembrances take up the mind space. In their rapid passage through the mind, you may not even be aware of each one, yet the painful impact of their contents can harm your self-esteem and cause emotional pain. With curiosity and skill, slow the blades and let go of them at the same time.

• *The somatics of yoga express the truth that thoughts can also be lodged in the body. Revisiting the thoughts can instigate a feeling reaction to them.* The pains of the past get lodged in the body. *Asana* may have released some of these buried feelings. Later, relaxing in meditation can actually bring these painful memories or feelings to the surface and distract us. Acknowledging them for investigation at another time and then letting them go can bring the focus back to the meditation practice.

- *A traditional way of soothing and centering the mind is to concentrate on the breath. Find a steadiness in breathing and you may find steadiness in the qualities of the mind.* The breath practice is a way to find a single point to focus on and draw the mind inward, to anchor it and come into meditation. Calming the mind is the gateway to calming the emotions.

- *When the mind chances upon feeling tones in the body, it may follow the memories of these feelings. Take note and move away from these thoughts.* As addicts we were sense-addicted in many ways. That was the point of the addictive process: to *feel* one thing and to *avoid* feeling something else. All conditions related to the senses and letting go of them can be a challenge—a practice to be taken up again and again as needed. Practice letting go of holding on: to perfection, to the silence, to lack of input—whatever the challenge is. Let it go.

- *It has been said that the mind can only think one thing at a time. That may or may not be true, but with practice we can choose the one thing we focus on and then, with practice, we can let it go.* We busy-brain addicts have experienced planning the future while regretting the past, and at the same time actively doing something and being impatient with it. This is the challenge: Do one thing at a time; think one thing at a time. Don't resist thought, just practice slowing the mind down by naming the thought, identifying its type, and then letting the thought go, dissipating it like a cloud. Concentrate on that thought without becoming seduced into its full story. Just think it and let it go. Now, one thought at a time allows you to choose.

- *A way to move away from concentrating on thoughts is to move away from naming and identifying thoughts, ideas, and the content* of the thoughts. As you find yourself seeing, classifying, choosing, or engaging in the thoughts, pause, and let the thoughts go. No judgment or criticism—just notice and let go. When we move deeper into meditation, the consciousness of thinking moves aside. This is a magical, unconscious process. Thinking about not thinking is a dead end. Just as you can't make yourself fall asleep, you can't make yourself not think. You find that this freedom from thought has happened when you "return" and start thinking again. You notice that you had not been thinking consciously a moment ago. Relax, don't chase it; let it go.

• One thing leads to another. As you find a train of thought, let it go. If the thoughts are resistant to being let go, then replace the unskilled or unhealthy thought with another, more positive and healthy one. Then let it go. If you are stuck in *samskara*, in the ruts of unuseful thinking, take this time to build new associations. Allow the mind to find the initial unhelpful thought and reframe it.

It can be helpful knowing the ways the mind can be distracting and distracted, knowing that we are all subject to this wild, galloping, turbulent, inquisitive, and repetitive mind. If meditation does not happen easily or regularly for you, then you are in good company. It is the practice that is so important. As my friend Stephanie Tate says, "If you have to call your mind back one hundred times, that is perfect. The only way not to do it right is not to do it."

SAMADHI: BLISS DIVINE

"*Samadhi* means moving into a sense of wholeness and balanced awareness,"[3] writes Mark Stephens. T K V Desikachar states, "When we succeed in becoming so absorbed in something that our mind becomes completely one with it, we are in a state of *samadhi*."[4] From reading these two quotes, I can say that I have had glimpses of *samadhi*. Let me elaborate: I am a potter. There have been occasions when I was so involved in "throwing a pot" that I heard nothing, was aware of nothing else but the clay spiraling beneath my hands. I have experienced that moment in nature—watching a sunset or sunrise, or when my concentration is absorbed in wonderment at the smallest bud opening on a flower or tree, or doing household chores like stirring something on the stove when all I am doing is stirring something on the stove; all is right with the world, and the only moment is now. Gazing into a loved one's eyes in a moment of total caring and selflessness can bring this timeless feeling of wholeness and union. Singing with a deep reverence, laughing out loud with sheer joy, or losing oneself in the action of artistic creation can give one that transcendent peek at *samadhi*. Stringing together these harmonious moments can inspire us to continue doing those things that bring us home—home to the true self, that contentment in union with our Higher Power and all of creation.

This final limb on the royal path, *samadhi*, describes a deep and profound state. This phase of enlightenment comes as the result of the other seven limbs being practiced with great skill. The other limbs are required to bring us to a state of enlightenment. This is a lifetime journey, or one of many lifetimes, as the Hindus would insist; it is of great interest and allure but it is fleeting except when achieved by the most skilled practitioner.

Further writings on this subject can be found in myriad classical yoga texts. We in the twelve-step programs discuss the difference between "having recovery" and "being recovered"; I take the position that I am "living in recovery," so my search for bliss divine continues. Each day that I am present and in the moment with someone in the program,

I am practicing the principles of yoga. I let outside disturbances fall away; I listen with focused concentration; I leave off planning my response; I hold that person in my total attention, finding our similarities and the union of our spirits, and this brings me to the experience of my new way of thinking, of health and healing. My recovery is kinetic; it deepens and progresses as I grow and become more authentic, more genuine. *Samadhi* is not a static destination; it is a part of the road ahead. The journey itself transforms me.

EXERCISE

BREATH-FOCUSED MEDITATION PRACTICE

Bring a timer of some sort to your meditation area.

* Sit in a comfortable position, on the floor or on the floor with the back against the wall, or on a chair with the spine erect in a way that you can maintain for ten minutes or more. If seated on the floor, you may find that a firm cushion under the buttocks can lift the hips sufficiently that the legs and hips feel more at ease. Once you are comfortable, set the timer for the amount of time you wish to sit in meditation, possibly ten minutes or more.

* Close the eyes, having them remain soft behind the eyelids. The eyebrows and muscles around the eyes are soft.

* Begin practicing the three-part yoga breath, first bringing the breath to the belly for three rounds, then to the belly and the ribs for three rounds, and finally into the full three-part breath— belly, ribs, and chest. Continue to breathe in this conscious way smoothly and slowly for several rounds, expanding the belly and then the ribs, lifting the chest. Exhale in reverse order: chest, ribs, and finally contract the belly slightly, expelling all the breath.

* Become aware of the ankles/feet against the ground, the legs on the surfaces they touch, and bring the awareness to the hips, to the belly, and back to the shoulders. Take the awareness from the fingers, hands, and wrists up the arms to the shoulders. Feel the collarbones soften, the throat soften, and the face soften. Let the forehead, eyebrows, and eyes remain soft. Breathe.

* Become aware of the breath either at the tip of the nose or at the center of the belly, somewhere in between, or at the back of the throat. Come back to this space when the mind wanders. Be aware of the temperature of the inhale at the tip of the nose and the temperature of the exhale. Allow awareness of the surrounding environment to slip away. If sounds, activity, or breezes call your attention away, bring it back to the breath. Inhale and exhale— slow and steady, deep and smooth, without any jerks or pauses. Continue to anchor yourself to your breath, dismissing those interesting thoughts with the word *later*. You can return to them later. Let go of judging the current experience. Come back to the breath. Invite the planning of the future to wait until "later," and allow the remembering of the past to wait until "later." Forgive the mind travel and return to the present.

* All that is important is this now, this moment, this breath.

* Continue to bring your mind back to the breath; keep practicing a breath at a time until the timer signals. Take a few deep, mindful breaths before opening your eyes and moving.

CHAPTER NINE NOTES

[1] Stephens, Mark. *Teaching Yoga: Essential Foundations and Techniques.* Berkeley, CA: North Atlantic Books, 2010, p. 101.

[2] White, Ganga. *Yoga Beyond Belief: Insights to Awaken and Deepen Your Practice.* Berkeley, CA: North Atlantic Books, 2007.

[3] Stephens, op. cit., p. 267.

[4] Desikachar, T. K. V. *The Heart of Yoga.* Rochester, VT: Inner Traditions, 1995, p. 109.

CHAPTER TEN

The Gunas and the Mind States

WE HAVE NOW MOVED INTO A more esoteric part of the recovery and yoga journey: the intersection of the steps, working the program, and the less well-known yoga concept, *gunas*. The *gunas* are the three basic states or qualities of energy of which all things are composed. In classical physics, we would call them solid, liquid, and gas. *Tamas* (solid), *rajas* (liquid), and *sattva* (gas) are the aspects that are said to make up all matter, emotion, and being, and their expressions and actions can be traced to one or another of the *gunas*. As an example of *gunas* in matter, take food: fresh, light, and juicy foods are *sattvic*; bitter, salty, hot, or dry foods are *rajasic*; and old, processed, or reheated foods tend to be *tamasic*. Music and sound, movement and dance, books and words, even seasons and times of the day evince one or more of these qualities. Various stages of recovery can be identified by their *gunic* qualities, and these will be explored later in this chapter.

• *Sattva* is the state of harmony and purity.

• *Rajas* is passionate, changeable, mutable. It is a very active state, moving between *sattva* and *tamas*.

• *Tamas* is dullness or ignorance. It is a heavy, dark state that is bound by inertia.

Durga Leela of Yoga of Recovery describes these three states in her course materials by drawing a mountain lake. In the *sattvic* mind, the lake is still and clear, reflecting the surrounding scenery, mountains and trees, shore and sky, with precision. Reality to a *sattvic* mind is clear and accurately reflected as well. When the lake is subjected to winds and rain, the surface becomes ruffled, and the reflection of the countryside around it becomes wobbly and somewhat distorted. So, too, with the impact of emotions and passions, with feelings and with fears, the world is somewhat unclear to the *rajasic* mind. When the lake is affected by tumultuous weather, with fierce rain and high winds, the lake becomes totally disturbed, and the sediment at the bottom is stirred up and blended with the water. The lake itself becomes totally murky. There is no reflection; even the moon in the sky does not light the lake, and there is nothing to be seen. The mind in deep states of denial, in torpid disassociation from reality, resembles the lake in its *tamasic* state. We in recovery would call this state our "bottom." While there are lesser experiences of a *tamasic* state, coming to grips with our addiction is the most profound one we can have. In fact, due to the sedentary (sedimentary) nature of this *guna,* a spiritual experience, or divine intervention, was needed to bring us into the *rajasic* state needed to be willing to change. Even in recovery we can experience *tamas* when we are in the extremes of greed, fear, self-righteous anger, resentment, and other less-than-lovely states. Often we cannot see our own *tamasic* state until we are in a meeting, hearing our truth in the story of another. We can experience a moment of clarity when reaching out to a sponsor or wise advisor who will lead us to see our own *tamasic* state, and thus we begin to move into *rajas*.

Rajas is changeable, active, and mutable. It is a comfortable state in modern Western culture, where doing more is being more. We double up appointments; we double-book ourselves; we multitask and work beyond our healthful capacity, fueling ourselves with caffeine and sugar and believing the busiest person is the most valuable person. Our culture supports these qualities by encouraging these values and promoting quick fixes to everything from states of being to states of mind, as well as physical conditions and attributes: quick teeth whitening, quick weight loss, in-and-out shopping, fast-food eating opportunities. The list is endless. In this fast-paced, do-it-now, have-it-all culture, it is no surprise that ACTION is a conventional and comfortable state. While there is no problem with mindful action, any action for the sake of motion alone is seldom healthful. *Rajas* is also a passionate state, often coming from immediate need without the use of much discernment. It is not a negative state per se; however, *rajas* is best experienced as a temporary state as one moves through it into *sattva*, or one can regress and fall back into *tamas*.

Sattva is the state of harmony, bliss, balance, and creativity. It is a calm state of equanimity. This is the state where life is seen in the right size and shape accurately, and responses are wise and proportional. This is the "fourth dimension" we talk about in the program—those moments when we are "happy, joyous, and free," and those rare days when we feel all the promises of recovery. *Sattva* itself is not a steady state, either. It is an experience in life and a condition to which to return time and again on our life's journey.

The *gunas* are not stable conditions. We move between and amongst them constantly. Our whole being is not fully one *guna* or the other. It is the nature of things to be mutable; how long an aspect remains in one *guna* or another depends upon one's spiritual fitness. In a connected state, one can veer more in the *sattvic* direction; in a recalcitrant frame of mind, *tamas* might be the prevailing condition. *Rajas* can be a state of change that moves in either a positive or negative direction. Considering the changeable nature of the *gunas*, different moments can elicit different experiences of them. I find myself more *sattvic* when seated in a recovery meeting, when I am preparing for a yoga class, or when I meditate. The next moment my mind can race ahead to things I need to do in the future or delve into self-recrimination for something I had not but should have done (*rajas*). I can even sink into a state of denial, being unaware of what troubles me, unable to see things clearly yet overcome with a sense of doom. This is a *tamasic* state, and often only a powerful moment of inspiration will bring me out—a dream, a sound or song, or an awareness brought about through meditation. Bringing the conscious mind into awareness of its condition is the first step in addressing it. Just as the first step in the program is admitting we were powerless over our disease, by identifying our condition and accepting it we can then begin the process of moving out of that condition.

I once had a very powerful dream about my son. I dreamt that he and I were walking on a forest trail. It started to rain, and to find cover I found us a burrow behind some tree roots on the hill next to the trail. He and I huddled there, and the rain continued unceasingly. As more rain poured down, the hillside began to wash away, exposing more roots. After quite some time in this burrow, trying to wait out the continuing storm, my child became hungry. I came up with the idea of making a soup with the rainwater and the newly exposed tender roots. He ate and ate, but appeared never to get full. The roots themselves doubled in number, and wherever I took a snip, cutting off one root, two rootlets replaced it. Nevertheless, I kept making soup to feed him. The roots over the opening to the burrow became more and more dense and morphed into what looked like cell bars. I panicked and felt trapped. All at once, a voice came to me: "That which can cure can kill." I woke up in a sweat with the sure knowledge that I could no longer coddle my son; I was not "filling" him with the soup of care, but creating a jail for us both. In my dream I was able to see that which I had been denying: I had been in a *tamasic* state relative to my relationship with my son.

This dream was such a powerful lesson to me that I named it "Twisted Root Soup," and I recall it whenever I am stuck in a pattern of "helpfulness" that really is debilitation. I had been powerless over this behavior until I recognized it. I was then able to move through *rajas*—a period of awkwardness and change—until I became more harmonious and *sattvic* in my relationship with myself, my intentions, and others.

Not all activities are of the same quality for all people: for example, sitting quietly in contemplation and stillness might be *sattvic* for the antsy, go-getter type, while making plans and making phone calls and getting out of the house may be *sattvic* for the depressed person. It is important not to quickly judge which *guna* is being experienced or expressed (especially when taking the inventory of others), but to reflect in a mindful way what quality you are embracing with any action or choice you make.

THE STATES OF MIND

Our state of mind affects this selection process. According to yoga, we have three levels of the mind: the subconscious, conscious, and superconscious. The subconscious is the repository of all experiences, events seemingly unremembered. It also harbors the unconscious decisions we have made throughout life as a result of these experiences, emotional reactions unfettered by reason or discernment, and base emotions grounded in self. Whenever we have had a traumatic experience, there are parts of the events that we remember and many others that we do not hold in our conscious memory. These unremembered events can have a powerful sway over us. We have made decisions based on them while not being aware of their influence, and these decisions affect our current choices and behavior. Our feeling self solidifies around a concept such as "I can rely on no one but myself," or "dark-haired men are dangerous," or "I always make mistakes so I won't try anything new," and so on. We may not be aware of why we won't ask for help, why our heart races when we are alone in an elevator with a dark-haired stranger, or why we avoid trying new things.

The conscious mind has discernment and judgment; it reflects on the experiences and remembered actions and activities and makes selections. The conscious mind makes choices between identifiable options. For example, we become aware of our shortcomings and make a decision to act in a new or different way than habit might suggest.

The superconscious mind is healthy intuition. While the conscious mind will weigh variables and make choices, the superconscious mind draws in the infinite—beyond the consciously known and the unconsciously known—and it just knows. This is the mind we search for in the Eleventh Step, seeking through prayer and meditation knowledge of the divine's will. This is the mind that abides within the divine—the true self that we are all seeking. We tap into this mind in meditation, and we live here when we reach *samadhi*.

As we move down the path in recovery and go through our action steps (Four through Nine), we bring more and more repressed content from the subconscious into the conscious mind. As we learn to live in the present, let go of control and self-seeking, and move into service, what we learn and do becomes more automatic and part of our superconscious. Step work is vital to the progression of our mental health and spiritual growth.

Being conscious of the way the mind works and becoming aware of the *gunas*, this continuum of qualities and emotions, can help our decision-making process about how we act, what we choose to do, and who and what we choose to be around. A desire to remain moving with purpose from *rajas* (that active, fluid state) to *sattva* (the state of harmony) encourages me to stay with the "winners" in the program—those who walk the walk, and not just talk the talk. It encourages me to avoid events and situations that will agitate or overstimulate me without a safety net or a safe, wholesome person to encourage me. I would go to a comedy show in a nightclub with a sober friend, but not alone, and not with an active drinker. I enjoy rock music, but if I feel emotionally unstable, I choose softer, less *rajasic* artists to help calm my emotions and improve my outlook. Taking a walk is a useful way to address out-of-balance feelings; however, walking in a mall would be too stimulating, while a hike in the hills could bring me closer to my relationship with the divine.

As I move closer to my authentic self, I become more aware of what can throw me off kilter, put me out of balance, and distance me from my healthy self. When out of balance, I am not able to access the good in me or the truth in myself, and I am unable to provide sustenance to myself and my recovery and meet others where they are. I am unable to be of service to anyone from a disharmonious state of mind and spirit. Taking the time to reflect on the *gunas* and their properties is part of the discipline of being in the moment—the moment of choice. I choose to stop, look, and listen, then to move.

EXERCISE

EXPLORING THE *GUNAS.*

First read and complete the exercise that follows.

The table below illustrates the intersections of the *gunas* and the mind states. Try to take something from your own Fourth or Eighth Step, and see how you can "move" it from the *tamasic* subconscious classification through amends and growth to (possibly) a more *sattvic* response or reflection. In addressing my powerlessness over bad eating habits, I had to admit what I was doing before I could change it. First, I had to acknowledge that I wanted to make better food selections. Initially I had experienced denial. I had a series of events that woke me up out of denial: the numbers on the scale, a feeling of indigestion on a regular basis, and a sluggish digestive system. (Awareness brings about a move to *rajas*.) In an unhealthier approach, I tried to mask my feelings of hunger with tea, or to change how I was feeling with the stimulant of caffeine. Taking a wiser path and employing the wisdom of others, I spoke to friends, began to do some research, and sought some counseling. I made a decision to deal with my concerns in a healthy, holistic manner (now becoming more *sattvic*). With practice I eventually started to make good food selections; later, these came with ease and intuition. My tastes changed, and a wider variety of flavors, food types, and preparations became more desirable.

See the example below and then try one on your own.

GUNAS	MIND		
	Subconscious	Conscious	Super-conscious
Tamas (unhealthy delusion, darkness, and resistance)	Denial of unhealthy eating. Excuses, rationalization, and justifications.		
Rajas (motion, energy, movement)		Drinking coffee to "get things done" and to quell hunger. Later investigating options, hopping from one solution to another.	
Sattva (balance and harmony)		Deciding to approach a situation with spirituality and coming from a healthy point of view. Seeking wisdom from others.	Intuitively approaching a situation from a healthy point of view.

With the concept that there can be three levels of an activity—thinking, speaking, and doing—actions can be traced to one of each of the three *gunas*. Healing and self-care can mindfully be selected for a more *sattvic* way of life.

	ACTION SOURCE		
GUNAS	Thinking	Speaking	Doing
Tamas	Denial of core worthiness.	Using absolutes in negative phrases—"You always mess things up."	Polluting the environment.
Rajas	Impatient demands, living in the future, perhaps reexperiencing craving.	Talking on the phone while typing on a keyboard; gossip and unkind speech.	Listening to loud unsettling sounds/music; gossiping or telling exaggerated tales.
Sattva	Kind self-talk.	Encouraging words to others and self.	Listening to soothing music.

See what comes to mind for you and complete the following chart.

	MIND		
GUNAS	Subconscious	Conscious	Superconscious
Tamas			
Rajas			
Sattva			

Expanding from the concept that there are three levels in which an experience can be expressed, complete the table below with examples from your own life.

GUNAS	ACTION SOURCE		
	Thinking	Speaking	Doing
Tamas			
Rajas			
Sattva			

Now complete the *guna* quiz at the back of the book. How does this fit for you today?

CHAPTER ELEVEN

Ayurveda and the Doshas

FINDING HEALTHY PHYSICAL, EMOTIONAL, AND SPIRITUAL balance and well-being is a complicated endeavor. We start our recovery journey with a period of withdrawal from our addiction. This takes our total consciousness and energy. Whether we are withdrawing from substances or behaviors, or possibly a combination of both, the first few weeks or months are spent exclusively on finding out what daily life is like without this crutch. After this initial period, possibly when the "pink cloud" begins to dissipate, we become faced with other recovery challenges, and each of us brings forward different issues due to our unique natures, histories, and individual personalities. Each of us has our own way of approaching life in general and this new life in particular. Yet even with unique beings, there are some more common types, some themes of behavior. These may first be seen in the personalities of other people. For example, it is possible that you have noted some predominant personality types in meetings, and perhaps these mirror and approximate our own. You may have noticed those people who jump into the program with both feet, whose enthusiasm knows no bounds. These people embrace the program fully and without reservation. There are others who are more laid-back, who observe, contemplate, and assess before becoming fully involved. There are yet others who will "go along to get along," participating lightly before becoming engaged. There are also combinations of these three types.

Each of us comes to the program with our own history, baggage, needs, and expectations. We make these manifest according to our characters: the enthusiastic embracer, the contemplative assessor, the "fake it till you make it" person. Again, there will be a combination of these types of behavior in each of us, and possibly a slight change from one to the other from time to time, but we each have a preponderance of one of the types. Ayurveda has examined these characteristics and mapped them, not only through our behavior but through all our physical systems. Each of these three main character types has a name: vata, pitta, and kapha. Each body has elements of each, and each person expresses one or more to a greater degree.

Ayurveda, a Sanskrit term meaning "science of life," is the most ancient system of medicine in widespread practice today. The word ayurveda comes from two words: ayus, meaning "life," and veda, which means "knowledge." There is evidence that it has been in continuous practice for more than 5,000 years. The goal of ayurvedic medicine is to restore the body to health, which in ayurvedic terms means balance—mind, body, and spirit.

Health is also defined as "physical and mental well-being; freedom from disease, pain, or defect; normalcy of physical and mental functions;

soundness" (*Sushruta Samhita*, various sources). The Sanskrit word for health is *svastha*, which translates as "to be established in oneself." In yoga we refer to health as being balanced: body, mind, and spirit, to be one's true *atman*, or self. In recovery programs we talk about releasing all that prevents us from being of maximum service to ourselves and others. In this, the aims of yogic, *ayurvedic*, and recovery philosophies are similar: the paths are interrelated and mutually supportive. These three paths all direct us to find balance, to be whole, and to be genuine and true to our inner selves.

THE *DOSHAS*

Ayurvedic doctors or practitioners consider one's personal character traits when doing a health assessment and before addressing one's out-of-balance condition. How does one know what is out of balance unless the true center is known? The initial step an *ayurvedic* practitioner will take when working with a client is to have the client prepare a character, or *dosha*, self-assessment. Each *dosha* is associated with characteristic tendencies that facilitate a diagnosis for the physician or practitioner. *Ayurveda* looks at the energies in the body, the digestion, the sleep patterns, and the skin and hair for signs of health or dis-ease. Dis-ease (more than disease) is the condition of being out of balance in any facet of one's being: mental, physical, or spiritual.

The three primary *doshas* are *vata*, *pitta*, and *kapha*.

VATA TYPE

This *dosha* is composed of the space and air elements. The body tends to be slender (lightest of the three body types) with cool, dry skin and dry hair. *Vata*-predominant people are creative and quick to grasp new ideas, but are also quick to forget. *Vata* persons are characterized by unpredictability, enthusiasm, and variability in diet and sleep. They tend to have high energy in short bursts but tire easily and overexert themselves.

Vatas are prone to headaches, hypertension, anxiety, dry coughs, sore throats, earaches, insomnia, irregular heart rhythms, premenstrual syndrome, abdominal gas, diarrhea, nervous stomach, constipation, muscle spasms, lower back pain, sexual dysfunctions, arthritis, and nervous system problems.

Their addictions of choice would be anything that would reduce pain and insecurity. All addiction is seen primarily to be a *vata* imbalance, and *vata* people are highly prone to it.

PITTA TYPE

Pitta types are made of fire and water, are usually of medium build and strength, and are able to easily maintain their weight. They tend to be intense, short-tempered, sharp-witted, and passionate, and have strong digestion and appetite. *Pitta* people are orderly, efficient, assertive, and self-confident, but can become aggressive, demanding, and pushy. They are fairly predictable in their routines as they eat three meals a day and sleep eight hours a night. Generally, their complexion is fair or reddish, often having freckles, and their hair is usually fine and straight, tending toward blond or red.

Typical health problems include heartburn, ulcers, hot sensations in the stomach or intestines, insomnia, rashes or inflammations of the skin, acne, skin cancer, anemia, and gallbladder and liver disorders.

People with *pitta* as their primary *dosha* look to drugs and activities that stimulate them and keep them going.

KAPHA TYPE

Kapha is composed of earth and water. People who are predominantly *kapha* have a solid, strong, heavy body type and soft hair and skin, usually with large, soft eyes and a low, soft voice. They tend to gain weight easily and need a lot of sleep and warmth. *Kaphas* are usually relaxed, graceful, slow moving, and affectionate. They are forgiving, compassionate, nonjudgmental, and faithful. This *dosha* type has the most energy of all the constitutions, but it is steady and enduring, not explosive. They procrastinate and are slower to learn but have excellent long-term memories.

Although *kaphas* generally have a strong resistance to disease, they are prone to obesity, allergies, colds, congestion, sinus headaches, respiratory problems, atherosclerosis, and painful joints.

Downers, alcohol, muscle relaxers, eating, and other low-key activities describe the addictive tendencies of the *kapha dosha.*

All three *doshas* are present in all beings; however, each person has a native or original state of being reflected in a dominant *dosha* or *doshas*. Most people are "bi-*doshic*," evincing the characteristics of primarily two *doshas*. While there are ten possible combinations of the three *doshas* (*vata-pitta, pitta-kapha,* and so on, up to *vatta-pitta-kapha*), we are more unique than just those ten types.

In addition to the *dosha*, the *ayurvedic* practitioner will evaluate diet, lifestyle, the climate patterns in which you live, the environmental conditions (including pollution), what you do for work, and your relationships and family life as well as your stage in life. The full picture can become quite complicated. Considering the *doshas* specifically, an *ayurvedic* practitioner evaluates the individual in terms of his or her psychophysical constitution and seeks to assist the individual in finding ways to return to a balanced state. Diseases are seen through the lens of "being established in oneself": determining if a person is in a balanced state with his or her true self or not. The description or name of the presenting disease or malady is considered unimportant; its effects on the body, mind, and spirit are important. Bringing the mind and body systems back into harmony returns the person to wellness, into *svastha*.

HOW THE *DOSHAS* CAN MANIFEST

Finding my access to my *svastha* took me many years of searching and only came late in my recovery. Initially, just quitting using had a profound impact on my physical health. Later, I became concerned with improving my eating habits and those of my family. Exercise and fresh air became important. At some point my interest in physical exercise became nearly manic and I became out of balance once again. I was off center. Remember that *svastha*, or health, means being in harmony with our true nature. We know our true nature, but in our dis-ease we have forgotten it. "Forgetfulness is a devastating disorder. We modern humans have forgotten our roots, we have forgotten our gods, and we are now busily trying to forget our morals . . . we are severed from our source of compassion, and we forget how to empathize."[1] I had forgotten who I was and who I was meant to be. This began with a life of rushing ahead—trying to be something other than I was or am.

Personally, I jump headlong into things. I do little if any research on a subject before I plow ahead, making the best of any impediments as I find them. I have taken jobs with little knowledge of how to do them; I started a family with no thought about how I would feed or raise my children. I am the sort of person who, when unchecked, can barely wait for someone to define a problem before offering a solution. This comes from my characteristic reaction to events from my background.

I responded to the terror and uncertainty in my childhood by making order out of chaos in order to feel safe. I developed a "take charge" attitude. My sister became more studious and withdrawn, abhorring the new and unplanned by removing herself from it. My brother discovered rage. Why these differences? We had the same parents, same living circumstances, and, aside from birth order, really not much difference in home life. Each one of us three siblings is a different *dosha*. The *ayurvedic* view would be that our responses to our upbringings are different because our characters are different. As a teenager I found an immediate solution to the need to quell my tumultuous feelings. I found boys, drugs, and alcohol. I am an active person, so downers and sedatives did not attract me. I preferred stimulants and the party atmosphere that drinking provided. While I had friends who were laid-back and more comfortable with downers and others who seemed to go along with anything just for the fun of it—not particularly invested in one experience or another—my character needed stimulation. I was resourceful, quick to learn the "codes" of various groups, and I could pass for competent at work or school and was (initially) able to keep my home life together.

I suffered from insomnia most of my life—even when not drug-impaired. I suffered from a sluggish digestive system, had dry skin problems such as eczema, and suffered from anxiety, which eventually became a constant condition. While I have been in recovery many of these symptoms have abated in their severity; I still face them, however. It was meeting with an *ayurvedic* practitioner named Durga Leela that enabled me to understand that all of these symptoms were physical and psychological responses to my *dosha* being out of balance. These responses were to be expected from someone with my combination of *doshas*, and the reoccurrence of any of these was a signal that I was not in harmony. I am a *pitta-vata* combination with some *kapha* influences. Knowing this, I am now aware of how to balance myself when I begin to experience my negative personality traits, or become physically unwell. The tools I use, the remedies and foods I eat to lessen my out-of-balance condition, are not the same as those of my best friend in recovery. She is a different *doshic* type, and her remedies are slightly dissimilar. For example, I need to reduce my activities to calm my overactive *vata*, while she needs to engage in more activity to increase her sedated *kapha*. Finding one's *dosha* is another tool to use in fine-tuning your own personal health journey in recovery.

There are several online resources to determine your *dosha,* and a simple questionnaire is included in the appendices in this book. Knowing what to do with this information is best explored with a certified *ayurvedic* practitioner. To find one, you can contact the National Ayurvedic Medical Association (NAMA). In addition to working with your *doshas*, the practitioner will offer several healing modalities associated with the senses and the elements. The five *doshic* elements are air, ether (or space), water, earth, and fire, and the senses are smell, hearing, taste, touch, and sight. Each *dosha* is associated with an element or elements as well as a primary sense or senses. The senses are stimulated in various ways and are associated with each *dosha* as part of the healing process. Each *dosha* expresses itself differently when it is out of balance, and hence the rebalancing of each *dosha* is unique and specific.

YOGA OF RECOVERY AND THE *DOSHAS*

I attended a Yoga of Recovery retreat at the Sivananda Ashram Yoga Farm in California a few years ago. There I was introduced to *ayurveda* in detail and its direct relationship to recovery. Durga Leela led the retreat in which we all learned about the *doshas* and their influences on and relationship to the roads of recovery. We were also introduced to the Six Tenets of Yoga of Recovery. These are:

- Life is Longing,
- Life is *Prana*,
- Life is Relationship,
- Life is Sweet,
- Life is Love,
- Life is Progress.

Durga Leela elaborates on each of these, integrating *ayurveda*, yoga, and twelve-step philosophy. We were given the opportunity to do some one-on-one work with her, and I developed a much deeper understanding of why I handle situations in a certain way, why my body responds to health and harm in the ways it does, and what I can do to establish a program of prevention for myself. I later became a certified Yoga of Recovery counselor myself, having learned even more, expanding on what we had learned in the retreat about the Six Tenets and the three philosophies. I came away with a deep understanding of the interrelationships of yoga, *ayurveda*, and recovery, and it became one of the major influences on my work.

Durga Leela identified the impacts of addiction on the *doshas*. Here is a summary of a few of those associations.

Substance/ Behavior	*Dosha*	*Vata*	*Pitta*	*Kapha*
Nicotine	Attraction	Use of hands, control, calms anxiety.	Feeling of heat and being in charge.	Removes lethargy, promotes image of the "good life" and creature comforts.
	Physical Cost	Dehydration, lung damage.	Dehydration and lung damage, heat bad for the *pitta* system.	Least damaged by dehydration due to constitution, but lung damage cannot be avoided.

continued on page 168

Substance/ Behavior	Dosha	Vata	Pitta	Kapha
Alcohol	Attraction	Reduce fear and anxiety, for fun.	Increases intensity of activities, increases already heated *pitta*.	Use alcohol for stimulation. Of all the *doshas*, may be the most affected by sugar content of alcohol.
	Physical Cost	Dehydration.	Damage to liver, blood and metabolic systems.	Weight gain, bloating, liver damage and heart disease.
Amphet-amines	Attraction	Likes activity, action, being on the go.	Likes the intensity, the high level of activity.	Not very attracted to "uppers"; more to depressants and downers, but will use them.
	Physical Cost	Dryness, dehydration, kidney damage.	Burns out nervous system, damage to the eyes.	None specified.
Gambling	Attraction	Excitement.	Like the challenge, attraction is to "break the game," to win the process.	Greed—want to win the money/prize. Acquisitive.
	Physical Cost	Sleep deprivation, disturbed eating cycles.	Disturbed eating and sleep cycles.	Disturbed eating and sleep cycles.

To go further now and to combine the *gunas* from the last chapter with the *doshas*, expanding on the work of Durga Leela and including that of other experts such as Dr. David Frawley and Dr. Robert E. Svoboda, the following shows how the illness of addiction could express itself in the *doshas*.

Gunas	Doshas	Vata	Pitta	Kapha
Rajas		Fear, anxiety, feeling ungrounded, emotionally cold, extreme shifts in mood.	Resentment, aggression, anger, blame, aggressive language.	Attachment, seeking comfort and ease, wanting the easy way, dependent.
Big Book/ Basic Text Descriptions (per Yoga of Recovery)		RESTLESS	IRRITABLE	DISCONTENTED

The *rajas* state for the *doshas* can be described as "restless, irritable, and discontented." Each person's *dosha* expresses his or her out-of-balance condition in a unique way. Anyone who has had the opportunity to work with a newcomer may recognize these three conditions. There are people who come to you feeling flighty and anxious—their thoughts run all over the place. Others may be full of anger and blame—"If you had my problems you would use, too." They have more of an attitude of fault-finding. Yet another newcomer may be extra-needy, desiring extra comforting, wanting a miracle cure or, at least, someone else to do the heavy lifting in their early recovery. Some may have a combination of attitudes, but there is usually one that is more prevalent than the others. Coming from a healthy sponsor place, you can just let the feelings come and go, intuitively knowing that each person processes in his or her own fashion. Knowing a little about the *doshas* can give you another tool in understanding a person's character and give an idea about how to approach that person—those a little more self-aware can use these tools themselves.

You can see from this chart that the effect on and response of each *dosha* type is generally specific to that *dosha* and can lead to specific outcomes. This *rajas's* changeable active period can occur on the way down the path to full-blown addiction, as well as during periods of change and growth in recovery. As a toddler becomes willful and unpleasant when learning a new skill like walking, a change born of frustration in acquiring a new proficiency, so too can unpleasant feelings come up in a *rajasic* manner in times of positive change. These *rajasic* expressions can also be signs presaging a possible relapse. Care is to be taken when these feelings come up, whether the change is in a *sattvic* or *tamasic* direction.

Gunas	Doshas	Vata	Pitta	Kapha
Tamas		Harmful to themselves, self-destructive behavior, cutting, suicidal tendencies.	Harmful to others, vindictive behavior, possible homicidal tendencies.	Stealing, manipulative, dependent/depressive personality, oversleeping, lack of motivation and drive.
Big Book/Basic Text Descriptions (per Yoga of Recovery)		HOSPITALS	JAILS	INSTITUTIONS

Durga Leela describes the addictive outcomes for the three *doshas* in the *tamasic* state as going to hospitals, jails, or institutions, as we say in recovery terms. The *vata* is most likely to end up in a hospital due to a breakdown of the physical systems and self-destructive behavior. The violent and antisocial behavior resulting in incarceration is most likely due to the expressive nature expression of the *pitta* part of a person. The dependent, passive attributes of *kaphas* lead them to be the most likely to be institutionalized.

The physical consequences of addiction manifest differently for each *dosha*. In the case of tobacco or marijuana addiction, a *vata* person may show symptoms of lung weakness, dry cough, and constipation, while a *pitta* person may experience infectious diseases of the lungs, liver, or blood. A *kapha* person, who has a more "moist" constitution, may show the fewest symptoms of all.[2] It is in the withdrawal stage that the *kapha* may have more distress.

SENSE THERAPIES AND MOVING INTO HARMONY

Sense therapies can help bridge the gap from the effects of "forgetting our true nature" (becoming out of balance) to embracing the fullness of our true selves (*svastha*). These sense therapies are ways to nourish and nurture ourselves. They are selected to decrease the overactive *dosha* (a flagging or low *dosha* is not seen as being powerful enough to cause problems).[3] As we are affected by all of our senses—sight, smell, taste, touch, and hearing—we can enrich ourselves by utilizing stimulations of these senses. While stimulation can be negative or positive, knowing these qualities can help us choose. For example, when you are feeling nauseated, the smell of food can be very off-putting, while to a person not experiencing nausea, the aroma of cooking can stimulate the appetite. Loud music can be uplifting or it can be disruptive. Knowing when to listen to it is the key. Listed below are some ways to calm an overactive *dosha*. These therapies can be used in a plan of self-soothing, as an adjunct to working with a sponsor and doing the steps, or with other forms of self-care such as *hatha* yoga.

In recovery I had to learn new ways to take care of myself, to spend time on myself. I had previously spent plenty of time scoring, drinking, sitting in a darkened room, and escaping life. In my step work, I finally admitted that I was not this selfless paragon, dedicating myself to survival and the maintenance of my family. Most of my energies had been spent in destruction of self. I now needed to put this energy into active self-care. This included attending to all of my senses. I was quite focused on taste, as I had earlier drunk so much. I found healthier ways to satisfy my taste and to calm my overactive *vata*. In fact, most substance addicts have a *vata* imbalance. Many *ayurvedic* practitioners concentrate on addressing and improving the balance of the *vata dosha* in order to help the addict gain health.

Alcohol is full of sugar; a look at the carbohydrate count on a wine label will confirm this. Now that I no longer drink, in order to satisfy my need for something sweet I look to nature to provide a substitute. When I first I got into recovery, I ate candy—lots of sugar candy. Now I eat fruit to take the place of sweets, and it satisfies my sweet tooth. This urge for sweets is still with me, so I keep fruits handy. To satisfy my need for stimulation, I put interesting things on the walls to busy my eyes; I listen to music (all types), and I have found that periodic massages bring my body into balance, as massage keeps the lymph moving and restores me to a calm state. I have chosen sense therapies that suit my personal inclinations in order to correct imbalance. I am aware both that I need this self-care and that it helps me stay in harmony with my true self.

To Heal the Senses	Dosha (examples of sources)	Vata	Pitta	Kapha
Smell	Flowers, incense, oils.	Sweet, warm, calming and cleaning: ginger, cinnamon, cardamom.	Cool and sweet: lavender, rose, jasmine.	Light, warm, stimulating: rosemary, sandalwood.
Sight	Paintings/art, pictures, flowers, nature.	Bright colors: gold, orange. Calming colors: blue, green, white.	Cool calming colors: white, blue, green.	Bright colors: gold, orange. Stimulating colors: yellow, red.

continued on page 173

To Heal the Senses	Dosha (examples of sources)	Vata	Pitta	Kapha
Taste	Foods, liquids.	Rich and nourishing foods: salty and sour tastes with moderate use of spices. Fruits, lightly cooked vegetables, grains except corn or rye, fewer beans; dairy and nuts are good.	Food that is neither heavy nor light: sweet, bitter and astringent tastes. Only cooling spices like fennel, turmeric and coriander. More fruit, vegetables. Avoid astringent foods like tomatoes, grapefruit, and cranberries. Add whole grains, but fewer nuts and oils.	Light diet with pungent, bitter and astringent tastes with liberal spices. Occasional fasting when appropriate. Eat artichokes, broccoli, and eggplant. Avoid grains, sweets, dairy products, and nuts.
Sound	Music, sounds of nature, chanting.	Meditative: To balance the volatile energy of *vata*, warm, grounding sounds are ideal. Listening to Gregorian chants, New Age pieces, and Bach's cello compositions should quell anxiety or emotional turbulence.	Soothing: *Pitta* types who are feeling overheated and irritable will be calmed by sweeter tones, such as light jazz, gentle flute music, and nature sounds.	Energetic: Out-of-balance kaphas will benefit from listening to active music such as rock and roll, rap, passionate classical pieces, and music with a strong beat and melody. These can invigorate and dissipate lethargy.
Touch	Massage, self-massage with oil (*abhyanga*)	Gentle warming touch with oils like sesame or almond.	Cool, soft-to-moderate touch with cooling oils such as coconut or sunflower.	Strong, deep massage with dry powders or stimulating oils such as mustard.

Svastha, in balance; emotionally, physically, and spiritually

Big Book of AA (p. 133) (per Yoga of Recovery)	HAPPY	JOYOUS	FREE

When we are practicing recovery and have adopted a healthy lifestyle and outlook, the *doshas* then manifest the Big Book descriptions of Happy, Joyous and Free. In choosing a style of yoga to help balance your *doshas*, you may need to take a careful look. Each *dosha* responds to a specific style of yoga better than another. It may seem counterintuitive, but to bring an out-of-balance *dosha* back into balance you may need to choose a style, just for that day or number of days, that is not the one you might be attracted to. So if you are experiencing too much *kapha*, you may be attracted to a restorative slow class when you might really need a more active practice. The following chart may help identify the various practices directed to calming the overactive *doshas*.

Doshas	*Vata*	*Pitta*	*Kapha*
Yoga to calm the Dosha	Slow meditative practice	Gentle vinyasa or restorative	Vigorous movement
Example asanas	Mountain pose Tree pose Child's pose Plow pose	Twists Seated forward folds	Sun Salutations Backbends Inversions

When bringing yoga into your self-healing practices, the *asana* and style choices can bring calm or can exacerbate a feeling of dis-ease, anxiety, anger, or lethargy. This is not to suggest that you need only to follow one type of practice, but that in a severely *rajasic* or *tamasic* time, the choice of one type of class could be more beneficial than another. It is an additional tool to use in times of stress. A balanced practice of moving through all types of poses in a proper sequence, with a calm and focused mind and a calm and focused breath, is the most beneficial way to stay in health.

The *ayurvedic* concept of health is found when body, mind, and spirit are in balance, when all aspects are working together in perfect union.

EXERCISE

Take the *dosha* quiz on page 196. Be as honest as you can be. If you are comfortable, share it with your sponsor. Without judgment, take a look at your step work and see if knowing your *dosha(s)* helps you to understand the themes and choices you have made. This is only a tool, a way of examining your past inclinations, "defects," and "shortcomings" in another light. See if you can identify some sense therapies you can incorporate into your life when you become out of balance. What could be used to prevent going out of balance? What type of *hatha* yoga practice might you try when feeling down or out of sorts?

CHAPTER ELEVEN NOTES

[1] Leela, Durga. "Yoga of Recovery" workshop materials, Sivananda Ashram Yoga Farm, http://www.yogaofrecovery.com/.

[2] Svoboda, Robert E. *Prakriti: Your Ayurvedic Constitution*, Second Edition. Silver Lake, WI: Lotus Press, 1998, p. 6.

[3] Ibid., p. 8.

[4] Frawley, David. *Ayurvedic Healing: A Comprehensive Guide*, Second Edition. Silver Lake, WI: Lotus Press, 2000, pp. 341–343.

CHAPTER TWELVE

Bringing It All Together

THE ROAD TO RECOVERY IS TAKEN one step at a time. A program of physical recuperation and integration is incorporated one step at a time as well. Whether you come to yoga early in recovery and avail yourself of the peace-inducing breath practices, mind-calming meditation, and detoxifying elements of the physical poses, or you come to it later in recovery to avail yourself of all these benefits as well as the mindful reknitting of your body, mind, and spirit, you do so one practice at a time.

As mentioned, addiction is a holistic disease affecting the emotions, mind, body, and spirit, so the healing must take into account all these aspects of our being. The twelve-step program addresses the emotions, the mind, and the spiritual aspects of recovery. Yoga and *ayurveda* also address the physical recovery. Controlling the breath, the ability to relax completely, the invigoration and energy releases of *hatha* yoga, and the five-senses therapies of *ayurvedic* treatments bring a completeness to the recovery model. The body has seen much harm and has suffered long neglect in the addictive life. Whether the addiction was to drugs or alcohol, with their toxic impacts on the brain and body, or to Internet browsing, sex, gambling, or unhealthy codependent relationships of any kind, the cost to the body in terms of tension, anxiety, poor sleep, and the devaluation of self-care has been great.

It is tempting to do it all now, to do it all together, combining all that yoga and *ayurveda* have to offer with all the suggestions of your recovery program in the hope of finding a mind-blowing immediate change and improvement of your well-being. However, it is suggested that you move slowly. You will see improvement, and it will come steadily as you incorporate each of the tools mindfully—letting the practices meet you where you are.

When I was new to my twelve-step recovery program, a gentleman at one of my regular meetings would go on about all the things he had to do in recovery, complaining that it was a full-time job. He would say, "I have to go to meetings, starting with ninety meetings in ninety days, and then go to several meetings a week from then on. I have to read the book, get a service job, work with my sponsor, do the steps, and then work with others. I won't have any time to LIVE!" Well, it may seem that way at first—the list of suggested activities early in recovery can be quite overwhelming. However, as I recall, the process of getting money to cop drugs or buy liquor, lying at work, recovering from benders, making excuses to everyone, and having scrapes with the law all took quite a bit of time as well. The road to health, consciously taken, does take time, and is more than worth the effort.

ONE DAY AT A TIME, ONE PRACTICE AT A TIME
Rather than being overwhelmed with all the practices, begin by adding some *hatha* yoga classes to your weekly schedule, hopefully

ones that also provide some breath coaching, which can be a gentle reentry to physical well-being. Yoga is a way to detoxify your body as well as a way to develop self-knowledge by becoming more acutely aware of your physical state. Conscious breathing practiced during a yoga class is a tool for staying in the moment and can be carried into everyday life to help monitor negative self-talk. Become aware of how you feel on the yoga mat, how you enjoy and incorporate the teachings, and see if this information about yourself can provide insight into how you are in life—bringing your experience from inside the yoga studio outside into your day. No need to practice each and every day, but a steady practice, a few times a week, will provide steady benefits. As regular attendance at recovery meetings adds to the totality and richness of your recovery skills, so, too, regular yoga practice adds to your treasury of unifying body, mind, and spirit experiences.

It may seem that all the varied yoga practices—developing the love of getting to know your Higher Power (*bhakti* yoga), learning about yourself and learning to love yourself (*jnana* yoga), maintaining mindful service to others without attachment to the action or its outcome (*karma* yoga), and the way to get there (the eight-limbed path of *raja* yoga)—will rob you of family time, hobbies, and entertainment. Nothing could be further from the truth.

Bringing yoga into your life does not have to be a complicated process. It can have a simple beginning, and be as basic as refining an intention or purpose for what you do, bringing consciousness to an ordinary act. For example, waking your child could include a moment in the doorway, feeling gratitude and love, before waking him or her for the busyness of the day. Taking the time to infuse that moment with love and compassion is yogic. Another example is adapting the focusing and centering slogans at meetings, like "To keep it you have to give it away," into types of yoga. These not only are foundational sayings of recovery, but also reflect a part of *karma* yoga. You can consciously identify the parallels between working the steps and the *yamas* and *niyamas* as you practice these principles. Finding mindfulness in what we do from the moment we step out into the world each day is a yogic tool. This can be saying a prayer or setting an intention for the day, such as practicing patience or "being of maximum service to those who still suffer." Meditating and clearing the mind for the possibilities of the day—doing what is in front of you and staying in the moment—are all tools that span both the eight limbs of yoga and the practice of the Twelve Steps. To further incorporate what yoga adds to your life, you can make it a habit to mindfully stretch your body a bit before you launch into the day. You could even do a yoga pose or two. Breathe. Eat a nutritious and appropriate breakfast mindfully, maybe keeping voice low and stimulus minimal as you start your day. Plan for sufficient time in the morning so the day does not begin in a noisy rush . . . and so on. Take care of yourself, your surroundings, and your family in the best way you are able. These simple acts bring yoga into your life.

The self-care techniques of *ayurveda* can be incorporated almost seamlessly into your daily routine. Merely adapting your choice of music to enhance your healthy mood, substituting oil for lotion for your skin, or selecting one vegetable over another (in accordance with your *doshic* needs) in the evening meal can be simple ways to mindfully include the balancing of your *dosha*.

People who have been in the program of recovery for a while will tell you that the principles of the program and the steps have become a part of their lives. It no longer seems like an effort to apply them, because the principles have become second nature. After your initial time of working through the steps, reading the recommended literature, becoming familiar with your Higher Power, and developing your meeting schedule, this work becomes part of your "spiritual tool kit." Working with others and with your sponsor becomes part of the rhythm of your days. Your yoga practice and *ayurvedic* self-care can be integrated in the same manner. It is just another set of recovery tools, a set of principles and activities that guide you to your best self, to the unwrapping and unfolding of your inner true self.

We change through the seasons of our lives, and so, too, our self-enlightenment journey changes and our self-care needs require reassessment. Each year, each phase of life—getting an education, having a family, being part of a family, dealing with aging parents, getting a love, losing a love, illness, aging, and death—offers unique challenges and opportunities to get to know yourself in a new and deeper way. Having additional tools or another method to observe and investigate your reaction or adaptation to these changes and the finding of your authentic self is critical to a healthful progression of the evolving you. That each one of these opportunities, these life events, is helping to unveil the true you, your genuine self, is a grace. Reach for the tools of the program and the tools of yoga and *ayurveda* for assistance in this journey.

As with all newly acquired skills, they can feel awkward when initially applied. It may feel time-consuming and possibly cumbersome. Learning to reach for them and use them can be a challenge. Be kind. Bring the concepts of the *yamas* and *niyamas*, *hatha asanas*, breath work, withdrawal, contemplation, and meditation into your life slowly. Weave them in with the steps of recovery; they go together easily. The Twelve Steps and the eight limbs lead to the same place—union of your body, mind, and spirit in the work of your Higher Power and in thoughtful service to those who still suffer. The selfish mind, the addicted mind, is a dangerous place to be. We must let go of old ideas and make room for a new way of living: a self-less life finding the true self. We are less concerned with issues that appeal strictly to our egos and find more interest in things that are of service and for a common good. This is the goal of moving into bliss, and bliss is not selfish, but it is of the self, the higher self, that abides in union with all beings and all living creatures.

Each person will be drawn to a facet of yoga and what yoga can bring to him or her at different points in recovery. Some of my students have been so delighted to find breath practices to help them during the day to moderate feelings of panic, abate rage, remove frustration, or calm anxiety. This is the first thing I teach, whether to newcomers or people with extended lengths of recovery. Other people, distracted by outside concerns, will need the activity and heat of an intense *hatha* yoga practice to focus on the sensations of the moment. It's hard to focus your mind on eliminating self-talk if your body is tense and your emotions chaotic. Meditation may be the relief sought by others who want some tools to approach the Eleventh Step—seeking "through prayer and meditation to improve . . . conscious contact" (*Alcoholics Anonymous*, p. 59). A student who has been working with me for several years says the practice of yoga has allowed her to feel grounded in her body and to trust her feelings more. Through mindful repetition of self-affirming phrases, reframing the way she speaks to herself, she is developing compassion for herself and patience with her growth. One of the twelve-step recovery mottos is "Change is a process, not an event." This is true in all facets of self-growth and illumination.

FINDING YOGA AND CHANGING YOUR BODY, MIND, AND SPIRIT

I came to yoga at first to settle my mind. In addressing the question of why I was so inconsolable, I discovered the resources of my inner being. I slowly made friends with my core, and have found many more tools to incorporate my true self into my living experience. Taking the workshops and going on retreats with people who were on a similar path allowed me to find my solace and strength through the companionship of others on this journey. I have learned that each person comes to this yoga and recovery journey with his or her own questions and challenges. The teachings are broad enough to help us all.

Some of the disease, or dis-ease, of our addiction is a habit of negative self-talk. We keep playing old tapes, entertaining erroneous ways of thinking about ourselves and our abilities, and they have developed into ruts in our minds. Memories of painful situations can be easily triggered and cause old feelings and reactions to surface in a heartbeat. It can be automatic to go down a path of self-deprecation and recrimination rather than bringing to mind our new, healthier self-image. These ruts, or negative habits of the mind, are referred to in yoga as *samskara*. Like a well-trod path or a skip in an old-fashioned record, the mind follows these patterns if left unchecked. The afflictions of our past actions are recreated by thought patterns that need to be changed at a base level. This takes diligent effort and vigilant attention. It is a process. This cleansing of the negative habits of the mind can progress with practice and advance from the noticing of the negative thought progression to, ultimately, a true inner detachment from these afflictions, giving one a sense of inner peace. The development of an inner prayer, resolution, or intention (*sankalpa*) can be a method of resolving these *samskara* and finding habits of the heart that can better benefit the repair of the self. This is another practice of self-care that can return us to health.

It is challenging to get into a practice and discipline of physical well-being. There can be tight muscles, limited joint movement, and often injuries that need to be healed before a robust physical yoga practice can be adopted. Trauma, stored in the body, needs to be released. As the body begins to repair, healing of the emotions also needs attention. A professional counselor may need to be consulted in addition to your recovery sponsor, yoga/*ayurvedic* mentors, and spiritual advisor. Again, the combination of all three will effect the greatest and best-sustained journey to healthy self-discovery.

In addition to our physical bodies, our physical surroundings or environments need to be assessed. Clutter in the cupboards, in the house and in the mind, prevents us from finding a serene place for daily meditation and study. A life built around rushing and schedules can make healthy eating seem like a remote possibility. Ordering the salad rather than the burger at a fast-food place may feel like the best we can do about healthy eating. However, besides contributing to proper diet and nutrition, the ritual of eating at a table with family or friends is nurturing. Eating on your lap in a car on the way to somewhere else is not. Being conscious of these differences, and making even small improvements, is a kind of yoga. Clearing the clutter, choosing to do one fewer activity so that you have one more moment with your family in mindful communion, taking five minutes in the morning to reflect on nothing (no plans, no rehashing of the past, no fantasizing about "what ifs")—is called meditating. This is recovery and this is yoga.

Being aware of the choices you do have for balance in your life is both recovery and yoga. Using the tools of the program, such as "Let Go and Let God," is like the *yama* of nonattachment—*brahmacharya*. So, in fact, our life does not need to feel overwhelmed with all these healthful activities; living itself becomes a healthful activity. Conscious practice of "the principles in all our affairs" becomes customary. These practices become the first thing you reach for during periods of change and unrest, rather than a pill, fix, drink, person, or thing. Healthy eating, healthy activities, healthy thinking, and healthy emotions become the norm when the path to your authentic self becomes the goal.

To further the skills of balancing your *doshas* and moving toward your true nature, there are additional methods to learn, more tools to add to the tool kit. When you are out of sorts, when, even in recovery, you find yourself in need of closing down and recalibrating your center, there are practices you can do to "right yourself." When I move into a mental attitude or an acting-out space, I realize I need to close shop for repairs. I slow down, take some time for introspection, and reexamine my habits.

• Have my eating, sleeping, or digestive habits changed?

• Have I added activities or dropped self-nurturing disciplines?

• What has changed?

• How long have I been moving in this direction?

It is important here for me to remind myself about the routines I habitually drop. The first thing to go is meditation (too busy). Along with that, I usually find myself eating poorly—either eating too much, eating too little, or moving toward a single source of food—mostly toast on the go, or only juice. I am jamming too many activities into my days and becoming a person on the go, not really being or going anywhere. I get into emotional, spiritual, and then physical trouble. I need to do something to stop the downward spiral. To do that, I reach into my reservoir of self-soothing techniques, starting with attention to the senses. I have a list of things I like to do for myself that address the lack of balance I am experiencing in my *doshas*. I made this list when I was feeling well and in a mindful, self-loving space. I go to it when I am not. This is how I came up with it.

The majority of us are multi-*doshic* (have characteristics representing two or all three *doshas*). I know that I am *pitta/vata*. I made a list of what soothes my *doshas*, brings them closer to balance and harmony. I started with the five senses and found something for each that I could easily access or participate in, to bring consciousness to that part of me. To soothe my sense of smell, I would take a shower or a bath using soap and shampoo with the scent of ginger. This usually calms and inspires me. I ensure that I have some favored foods available, ones that ground me. I enjoy baked apples with raisins and cinnamon. I select gentle music and play it softly while I work. I reduce my activities, deferring until later what I can. I take time to meditate, and I move my body in some form of *hatha* yoga. Before sleep I make sure I use a pleasant oil and do some massage before turning off the light. Tomorrow will be a new day.

Almost every activity one can perform has variants—variations in performance that will either move one to the *sattvic* (harmonious) balanced state or aggravate and stimulate one. As an addict, and therefore innately "preferring" chaos, it took me time and practice to prefer calm and equanimity. I would previously have jacked myself up with loud music, drunk plenty of coffee, eaten a candy bar, and pushed myself through my day with anger and resentment as fuel. Now my choices are much wiser; I find sensory stimulation that brings me into composure.

Through the path of recovery and my recovery mentors, the study of yoga and my yoga teachers, and incorporating *ayurvedic* self-soothing techniques, I have found a way to enhance the spirituality of my recovery program with the spirituality of my yoga practice. I have also found that my yoga practice amplifies my relationship with my Higher Power in my recovery program. Hand in hand, practice by practice, and tool by tool, I have found a way to embrace my life and myself—on and off the mat.

EXERCISES

Using the information obtained so far, or from further readings from the bibliography, select categories and complete the chart below. Use the five senses as a guide and find at least one activity or process to address healing and balance your *doshas*.

Sense	Healing Activity/ Process	Vata	Pitta	Kapha
Example: (for *vata/pitta* combination) **Sight**	Watching movies.	Bright, light movies with rich images and colors; comedies or documentaries.	Calming story lines with soothing commentary.	N/A
Sight				
Smell				
Touch				
Taste				
Hearing				
Asana **Practice**				

EXERCISE

Practice *dharana* (ten to fifteen minutes), reflecting on what you have read. What is the most important part to you? Write it down and make a plan to practice this daily for ten days. What was your experience? If you desire, repeat this exercise and see what new concept or practice floats to the top. Practice this for ten days. And so on. It is not necessary to implement all you find interesting all at once. Doing a little at a time can result in a permanent change.

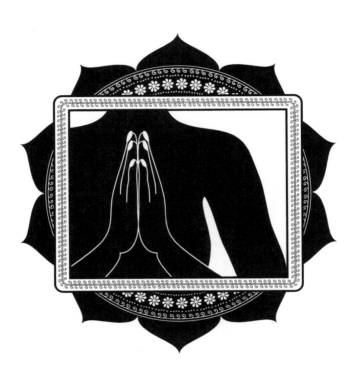

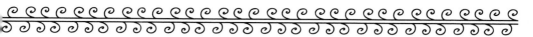

Styles of Yoga

ANANDA

This yoga practice is especially good for removing old, negative mind tapes. The affirmations can build a healthier repertoire of self-talk. Its focus on form and alignment engenders in the new yoga student a feeling of comfort and ease. *Ananda* yoga was developed in the 1960s by Swami Kriyananda. He had his training under Guru Paramhansa Yogananda, who wrote *The Autobiography of a Yogi*. In this yoga practice the instructors guide their students through a series of gentle *hatha* postures that focus on proper alignment, easeful posture transitions, and controlled breathing exercises (*pranayama*).

www.expandinglight.org

ANUSARA

Anusara is an integrated approach to *hatha* yoga with attention to the biomechanics of the poses. It is based on the belief that each person is equally divine in every part: body, mind, and spirit. *Anusara* focuses on three key areas of practice: attitude, alignment, and action. Founded by John Friend, this practice has had a rise in popularity in recent years. This is a good form of yoga for people in recovery who are looking for a vigorous practice.

www.anusara.com

ASHTANGA

Ashtanga was developed by K. Pattabhi Jois and is physically demanding, not designed for beginners. Participants move through a series of flows, jumping from one posture to another in order to build strength, flexibility, and stamina. This is a more athletic form of yoga and good for those who want to delve into the physicality of the practice.

www.ashtanga.com

BIKRAM

Bikram Choudhury, who sequenced a series of twenty-six traditional *hatha* postures to address the proper functioning of every bodily system, also incorporated a specific "climate" for the practice: heating the room to 104°. There is less attention on the form and alignment and more on the benefits of purification through sweat. This is a good practice for the experienced student who desires to detoxify from substances including nicotine, preservative-laden foods, and so on.

www.bikramyoga.com

HIMALAYAN YOGA

The purpose of the Himalayan Tradition is to awaken the divine flame within each human being, to know his or her true self. The *asanas* are taught with emphasis on mindfulness and self-observation. Yoga performed with this mindfulness allows one to refine the body and its movements, while learning to live in the present. Living mindfully and in the present is the finest way to live. This is the lineage I come from, and I wish to express deep gratitude to Sarla Walter and her student Kate Walsh. They have taught me selflessly and with infinite patience. This is the style I practice in all the locations where I teach. It is appropriate for all levels of recovery and all levels of skill on the yoga mat.

INTEGRAL

Integral Yoga is so named because the practice integrates everything—body, mind, and spirit. Classes also incorporate guided relaxation, breathing practices, *mantra*, and silent meditation. This is a very healthful practice incorporating all of the yogas in furtherance of self-awareness. It is appropriate for beginners and people at all levels of practice.

www.integralyogaofnewyork.org

IYENGAR

B K S Iyengar reigns as one of the most influential yogis of his time. His focus on the foundation and alignment of the poses set a new standard for teaching. The poses are held for a longer period of time in an Iyengar class. Attention is paid to the details of the pose and the biomechanics of the musculature and skeletal positions. Iyengar brought into common practice the use of props, including belts, chairs, blocks, and blankets, to help accommodate any special needs such as injuries or structural imbalances. These allow more poses to be available to more people in a healthful and safe manner. An Iyengar practice grounds the student deeply in the sensations of the body. This body awareness is a key step in developing awareness of the self.

www.iyisf.org

JIVAMUKTI

The *jivamukti* yoga method is a deeply philosophical and physical type of yoga, created by David Life and Sharon Gannon in 1984. Classes are developed along a theme (often *ahimsa*, or devotion). They include music, chanting, and *pranayama* in addition to the *asanas*. This is a wonderful tradition if you want to infuse *bhakti* yoga into your *hatha* practice.

www.jivamuktiyoga.com

KALI RAY TRIYOGA

Kali Ray (Kaliji) developed the Triyoga movements after having been inspired during a group meditation. There are several levels of adeptness, the first of which is slow rejuvenating practice supported by breath work. Meditation is a part of every class. This practice is deeply meditative, promoting relaxation and inner peace.

www.kaliraytriyoga.com

KRIPALU

The Kripalu Center for Yoga & Health has helped guide thousands of people along their path of self-discovery. Its founder, Amrit Desai, developed movements into three stages of practice, which he could then teach to others. These three stages are willful practice, willful surrender, and meditation in motion. Students may experience the release of emotions and internal thoughts during this practice with an experienced teacher.

www.kripalu.org

KUNDALINI

Yogi Bhajan brought *kundalini* yoga to the West, releasing it from its secret practice (it was originally practiced by a select few). Yogi Bhajan's point of view is based on the philosophy that it's everybody's birthright to be "healthy, happy, and holy." This yoga practice will detoxify mind and body and move you into and through your imagined limits. Classes are focused on *kriyas*, or sequences designed for therapeutic purposes. There is an important *kriya* about breaking addiction. You ball up your fist and place your extended thumbs to your temples, applying light pressure, at the same time locking the back molars and alternately releasing them right and left while internally chanting *sa ta na ma* for five to seven minutes and beyond. The thumb pressure sends a current of electricity into the central brain right under the pineal gland to balance it and send its pulsations to the pituitary gland, which regulates all the glands.

This is a very appropriate yoga style for people along all recovery paths.

www.3HO.org

POWER YOGA

Power yoga is adapted from *ashtanga* yoga. It is a series of poses designed to create internal heat and energy. It is a very mobile practice that may test your endurance. It may be practiced in a heated room. It is one of the types of yogas commonly found in gyms and athletic clubs. Some people may approach this as a purely athletic practice, enjoying the physical components. This style of yoga is useful for developing body awareness and presents an opportunity to practice your *yamas* and *niyamas* in your own personal practice, remaining aware of your own capacities.

SIVANANDA

This spiritually focused practice incorporates *pranayama*, relaxation, and *asana*. It uses primarily twelve foundational poses; less attention is paid to form and alignment and more to the transformative possibilities of the poses. The *sivananda* practice incorporates much more than *asanas*, promoting five main principles: proper exercise (*asanas*), proper breathing (*pranayama*), proper relaxation (*savasana*), proper diet (vegetarian), and positive thinking (*vedanta*) and meditation (*dhyana*). The chanting, *pranayama*, and meditation that are included are to help students release stress and blocked energy. The Yoga of Recovery was developed at the *sivananda* ashrams where retreats and trainings are held. This is a useful practice style for people in recovery, as it includes an investigation into the true self.

www.sivananda.org

VINIYOGA

Sri T. Krishnamacharya is the teacher of well-known contemporary masters B K S Iyengar, K. Pattabhi Jois, and Indra Devi. Viniyoga makes use of modified yoga poses that are designed to meet the specific needs of an individual and enhance healing, flexibility, and strength of joints. Viniyoga poses also intend to promote the feeling of well-being and strength. Krishnamacharya's son, T K V

Desikachar, continued this principle and developed the practice of Viniyoga. *Pranayama, dharana,* and *dhyana* can also be included, which can make Viniyoga a natural fit for some recovering people.

www.viniyoga.com

WHITE LOTUS

White Lotus yoga is the collaborative effort of Ganga White and Tracey Rich, who meld two eclectic backgrounds and years of experience into a nondogmatic teaching approach dedicated to helping students develop a well-balanced personal practice. Class formats may incorporate alignment, breath, and the theoretical understanding of yoga. White Lotus has had a profound impact on my practice.

www.whitelotus.org

HATHA

If you are browsing through a yoga studio's brochure of classes and the yoga offered is simply described as *hatha,* chances are the teacher is offering an eclectic blend of two or more of the styles described above. It's a good idea to ask the teacher or director of the studio where he or she was trained, if the poses are held for a length of time, if you will be expected to move quickly from one pose to the next, and if meditation or chanting is included. This will give you a better idea of whether the class is vigorous or more meditative.

Ayurvedic Resources

WHAT IS YOUR *DOSHA*?
WHAT IS YOUR *PRAKRUTI* (BODY CONSTITUTION)?

Circle the answers based on the state of your natural being throughout your life. The focus is you, the real you, not what happens to be true recently or what you wish to be. You may float between two answers; in that case, pick both. Add up the totals for each v, p, and k at the end. The results will tell you if you are *vata*, *pitta*, *kapha*, or any combination of the three.

1. PHYSIQUE

v) I am a slender person and I hardly ever gain weight.

p) I am of medium build.

k) I am well built and I gain weight no matter what I do.

2. SKIN

> v) My skin is dry and thin, and itches often.
>
> p) My skin looks flushed; I have lots of moles and freckles on my body.
>
> k) My skin is smooth and soft; it looks pale sometimes.

3. HAIR

> v) My hair is dry, thin, and brittle.
>
> p) My hair is neither dry nor oily (men: receding hairline).
>
> k) My hair is thick, full, lustrous, and slightly oily.

4. FACE

> v) My face is oval.
>
> p) My face is triangular (pointed chin, prominent jawline).
>
> k) My face is round.

5. EYES

> v) My eyes are small; they feel dry often and have a bit of dullness (usually brown).
>
> p) My eyes are medium in shape, and are sharp and penetrating (usually blue).
>
> k) My eyes are big and round in shape, with full eyelashes.

6. HANDS

v) My hands are generally dry and rough, with slender fingers and dry nails.

p) My hands are generally moist and pink, with medium fingers and soft nails.

k) My hands are generally firm and thick, with thick fingers and strong, smooth nails.

7. JOINTS

v) My joints are small, with prominent bones, and often crack.

p) My joints are medium and loose.

k) My joints are large and sturdy, with lots of surrounding muscle.

8. ACTIVITIES

v) I am a very active person (always on the go, mind constantly thinking).

p) I like to think before I do anything.

k) I am steady and graceful (I don't like to rush).

9. ACTIONS

v) I walk fast and talk fast.

p) My actions are very thoughtful and precise.

k) I like a slower pace and I take my time to accomplish things.

10. SLEEP

v) I do not sleep soundly at night. I tend to toss and turn. I wake up early in the morning.

p) I am a light sleeper, but if something wakes me up I can go back to sleep easily.

k) I am a heavy sleeper.

11. APPETITE

v) Varies; sometimes I feel hungry, sometimes not. I feel anxious if I don't eat.

p) I always feel hungry. If I don't eat I get irritable and angry.

k) I don't feel very hungry. I can go without food easily for a day.

12. BOWEL MOVEMENT

v) I tend to have constipation and can go a day or two without a bowel movement.

p) I am regular and sometimes stools are loose (tend to get diarrhea).

k) I have no problem. I wake up to go to the bathroom.

13. VOICE

v) My voice tends to be weak or hoarse.

p) I have a strong voice; I may get loud sometimes.

k) My voice is deep and has good tone.

14. EMOTIONS

v) I am a born worrier; I often feel anxious and nervous.

p) If things don't happen my way, I feel irritable and angry.

k) I am a happy person, very caring and loving.

15. WEATHER PREFERENCE

v) I love warm and humid weather.

p) I enjoy cool weather; I dislike a warm climate.

k) I like warm but dry weather.

16. SWEATING

v) I sweat a little but not much.

p) I sweat profusely and it might have an unpleasant odor.

k) I never sweat, unless working very hard.

17. MEMORY

v) I remember quickly and forget quickly.

p) I remember what I want to remember and never forget.

k) It takes me a while to remember, but once I do I
     never forget.

18. ACTIONS

v) I tend to be spontaneous.

p) I am a list maker. Unless I plan, I don't do anything.

k) I don't like to plan; I prefer to follow others.

19. STAMINA

v) I like to do things in spurts and I get tired very easily.

p) I have medium stamina.

k) I can work long hours and maintain good stamina.

20. MIND

v) My mind gets restless easily (it starts racing).

p) I get impatient easily.

k) It takes a lot to make me mad. I usually feel very calm.

21. DECISION MAKING

v) I change my mind often and will take time to make a decision.

p) I can make a decision easily and stick with it.

k) I want others to make the decisions.

22. PERSONALITY

v) "Can I change my mind?"

p) "It's my way or the highway."

k) "Don't worry, be happy."

23. SPORTS

v) I like action.

p) I like to win.

k) I like to have fun.

24. HEALTH PROBLEMS

v) My symptoms are mainly pain, constipation, anxiety, and depression.

p) I often get skin infections, fevers, heartburn, and hypertension.

k) I tend to get allergies, congestion, weight gain, and digestive problems.

25. HOBBIES

v) I like art (drawing, painting, dance) and travel.

p) I like sports, politics, and things that get my adrenaline pumping.

k) I like nature, gardening, reading, and knitting.

TOTAL: V (*VATA*)_____   P (*PITTA*)_____   K (*KAPHA*)_____

WHAT IS YOUR *GUNA*?

This particular test is derived from *Yoga and Ayurveda* by David Frawley (Dr. Vamadeva Sashtri). Fill in a cross for each section that matches your current position and then total each column at the bottom to see your current leanings.

GUNA/MENTAL CONSTITUTION CHART

Diet		Vegetarian		Some meat		Heavy meat diet
Drugs Alcohol and Stimulants		Never		Occasionally		Frequently
Sensory Impressions		Calm and pure		Mixed		Disturbed
Need for Sleep		Little		Moderate		High
Sexual Activity		Low		Moderate		High
Control of Senses		Good		Moderate		Weak
Speech		Calm and peaceful		Agitated		Dull
Cleanliness		High		Moderate		Low
Work		Selfless		For personal goals		Lazy
Anger		Rarely		Sometimes		Frequently
Fear		Rarely		Sometimes		Frequently
Desire		Little		Frequent		Excessive
Pride		Modest		Some ego		Vain
Depression		Never		Sometimes		Frequently
Love		Universal		Personal		Lacking in love
Violent Behavior		Never		Sometimes		Frequently

continued on page 204

Attachment to Money	Little		Some		A lot
Contentment	Usually		Partly		Never
Forgiveness	Easily		With effort		Hold grudges
Concentration	Good		Moderate		Poor
Memory	Good		Moderate		Poor
Willpower	Strong		Variable		Weak
Truthfulness	Always		Most of the time		Rarely
Honesty	Always		Most of the time		Rarely
Peace of Mind	Generally		Partly		Rarely
Creativity	High		Moderate		Low
Spiritual Study	Daily		Occasionally		Never
Mantra/Prayer	Daily		Occasionally		Never
Meditation	Daily		Occasionally		Never
Service	Much		Some		None

TOTAL: *SATTVA* _____ *RAJAS* _____ *TAMAS* _____

APPENDIX III

Asana Sequences and Guide

LIST OF *ASANAS*

While this list of poses and sequences is a useful home practice tool, it is no substitute for attending regular *hatha* yoga classes and obtaining guidance from a qualified teacher.

Here are some *asanas* that I teach in my classes.

One-hour to ninety-minute *asana* practice. (Reduce the number of repetitions to five from ten to practice a shorter amount of time. To get the full benefit of the practice, do not skip the breathing routine or the final relaxation. These are key to resetting the mind and emotions—to integrate the practice with the spirit.)

BREATH PRACTICE:

Coming into a tall-seated position, select one of the breathing disciplines and practice it for at least five minutes before beginning your *asana*. Before beginning the practice, set an intention—patience, acceptance, gratitude, or some other characteristic or value you wish to reinforce in your life.

WARM-UP SERIES:

Coming into quadruped and remembering to support the movements with the breath, move between cat and cow poses about three times.

Move to the tiger stretch/parallel balance sequence: extending the right leg behind you, toes flexed on the mat, lift the leg parallel to the floor (toes to the ground, knee toward the mat, and hip toward the mat). When you are balanced, extend the left arm in front of you directly out from the shoulder, thumb to the ceiling and fingers extended into the room in front of you. Return hand and knee to quadruped and repeat with the left leg and right arm. Repeat on both sides for a total of three rounds.

Downward-facing dog series begins from quadruped. Pushing into the hands and tucking the toes, float the knees a few inches above the mat. Breathe here for three to four full breath cycles. Return the knees to the mat. Again float the knees, and then, pushing into the arms, bring the belly to the thighs. Breathe here for three to four full breath cycles. Return the knees to the mat. Finally, float the knees, press the belly, then extend the heels toward the floor and breathe here for three to four full breath cycles. Walking the feet to the hands, move to forward fold.

Keeping the chin on the chest, pressing into the feet slowly, roll up to standing mountain pose.

To complete the warm-up, do some slow rotations of your shoulders, do wrist circles, and then clasp the hands behind you, raising the arms up toward the ceiling to stretch the front of the chest. Next, interlock the fingers, flip the palms forward, and raise the arms over the head to stretch the space between the shoulder blades. Proceed into the half-sun salutation and repeat it three times.

HALF-SUN SALUTATION:

Raise arms in an upward salute, bend back slightly, and come into a forward fold with soft knees; rise up halfway with hands on shins, looking forward and arching the back (monkey pose), and fold again, facing your knees. Rise up with flat back, winging arms out to the side; straighten into upward salute, follow with slight back bend, and return to *tadasana*, lowering the hands through prayer pose (*anjali mudra*) and returning the hands back to the sides. Repeat at least three more times, being conscious of the breath, timing it with the movements.

HEART OPENING SERIES:

Hold each pose a minimum of three complete breaths when you are able; extend to five if you wish.

Lunge (or modify by doing a half-lunge) two times per side, then move to lunge (or half-lunge), rotating the body toward the forward knee, repeating three times per side. Step into triangle three times per side, following with the pyramid pose with hands on hips, then pyramid with hands clasped behind back, repeating three times each side. Return to standing mountain and then step the right leg back for warrior II pose. Return the right leg to the top of the mat and step into the pose on the left side. Repeat three times per side, alternating between sides.

Take a few breaths in standing mountain, or *tadasana*, then lift the right leg into position for tree pose to balance. Return the right leg to the mat and repeat on the left side. Descend to the mat. Lie on your belly for cobra pose, lifting on the inhale and returning to the mat on the exhale. Do this three times, holding for two full rounds of breath on the third repetition before returning to face-lying pose. Roll onto your back for bridge. Hold in the extension for three to five breaths. Repeat this pose three times. Bring knees to the chest to release the pose. Roll onto your side and up into seated staff pose. Forward fold with soft knees. Breathe five full cycles here. Ease yourself back on the mat; draw the knees to the chest and come into a simple twist on each side, remaining in the twist for several deep breath cycles. Ease your way back into *savasana*. Remain here for five minutes or more.

POSE INSTRUCTIONS

Easy pose (*sukhansana*). Sit in tall, comfortable, cross-legged pose, balancing the shoulders over the hips, arms dropping down from the shoulders, hands on knees or in lap. Keep the spine tall but not rigid, the nape of the neck long, and the head balancing on the top of the spine. Allow the face, throat, neck, collarbones, and chest to

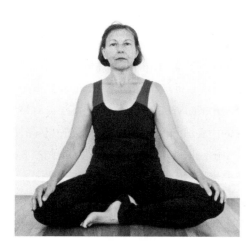

be soft. At the beginning of a yoga session, this is the pose to use to engage a breath practice. Begin one now and continue for a few moments. Set an intention for your practice before beginning to move.

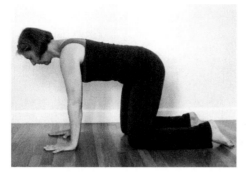

Hands and knees pose, or quadruped. Come to hands and knees, keeping the wrists under the shoulders and the knees under the hips, feet directly behind the legs, toenails on the mat. Using the abdominal muscles, keep the back flat and face the mat, pushing strongly into the mat with all the fingers and palms of each hand, the length of the shins, and the tops of the feet. This is the starting position for other poses.

Child's pose (*balasana*). Move the hips down toward the heels and reach the arms forward, opening up the chest. Rest your forehead on the ground. If the head does not reach the ground, stack the fists or use a prop to support the head. Breathe deeply into the belly and the lower back. Use the strength of the arms to come out of the pose. This is also known as the pose of wisdom; wisely choose this pose if you become fatigued in your practice, if your breath becomes raspy or ragged, or if you begin to hold your breath in effort. The breath will guide you; it will tell you the truth. If it does not flow freely, smoothly, and deeply, take a moment in child's pose and then return to the practice.

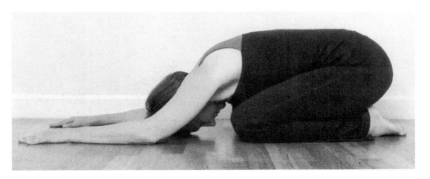

Cat/cow stretch (*marjariasana* to *bitilasana*). From quadruped, move into cow stretch; inhale, allowing the belly to drop, the chest to draw forward between the arms, and the hips to dip forward. Breathe a few rounds here. With an exhale, arch the back into cat pose, dropping the head to gaze toward the legs, tucking the hips under. Raise the middle back toward the sky. Breathe here a few rounds and, timing the next inhale, move smoothly into cow. Move back and forth between the two poses several times, perhaps in time with inhalation and exhalation. Come to stillness and rest.

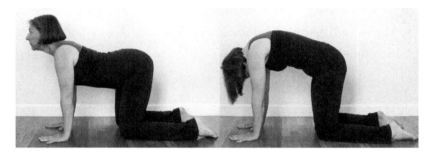

Tiger or diagonal stretch (*vyaghrasana* variation). From quadruped, extend the right leg back, keeping foot flexed, and hip, knee, and toes pointed toward the mat. Lift the leg level with the hip, parallel to the mat. Grounding the top of the left foot and shin onto the mat, raise the left arm up, stretching forward, parallel to the ground, fingers away from the body and thumb to the ceiling. Strongly extend the left arm forward and the right leg back through the heel of the right foot. Breathe three to five cycles of breath and return hand and knee to the mat. Repeat on the other side.

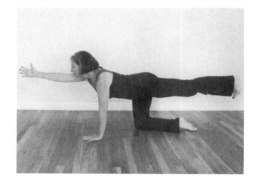

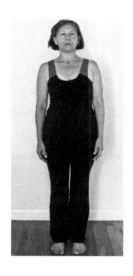

Standing mountain (*tadasana*). Standing tall with arms at your side, set feet parallel to one another a few inches apart. Make full contact with the mat/ground/globe with the soles of your feet. Feel the distribution of your weight and strive to make it even. Push down into the mat, rooting your feet to the earth, bringing that connection up through the shins. Raise the kneecaps and bring strength to the inner and outer thighs and the back and front of the legs. Tuck the tail, raise and grip the belly below the navel, soften the chest, lengthen the back of the neck, and drop the shoulders to the back, arms heavy and the head floating on the top of the spine.

Runner's lunge pose. From *tadasana*, bring the right leg back and bend the left knee directly over the ankle, hands on either side of the left foot, using a block or prop if the arms do not comfortably reach

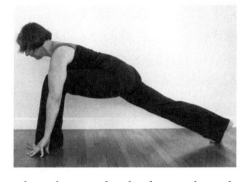

the ground. Maintain the length and strength of *tadasana* through the right straight leg. Allow the right foot to be strongly flexed and feel energy moving from the back right heel through the crown of the head. Breathe smoothly for several rounds. Return the right foot forward and switch legs. (Variation is to drop the knee of the back leg to the ground, using a blanket or doubled-up mat to protect the knee if it is sensitive.)

Crescent pose (*virabhadrasana* II, variation). From *tadasana*, bring the right leg back and bend the left knee directly over the ankle. Bring the arms up to the left knee and pause with the spine straight and chest opening. Raise the arms forward and then up over the head,

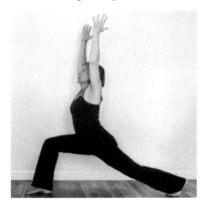

looking forward. Allow the gaze to look up toward the hands if the neck is loose and experiences no tightness or pain. Hold for several breaths, then return hands to waist before bringing the right foot forward to meet the left, returning to *tadasana*. Rest and repeat on the other side.

Pyramid pose (*parsvottonasana*). From *tadasana*, step the right foot back about three-fourths maximum stretch, facing right toes toward the front of the mat (possibly a forty-five-degree angle). Bring the arms behind the back, grabbing the right elbow with the left hand and the left elbow with the right. Pushing into the feet, draw up into the straightest standing pose available, and then, "hingeing" from the hips, fold forward over the left leg. Stay here for three to five full breath cycles.

Using the strength of the legs, come back up to standing, release the hands, and return the right foot to the top of the mat. Breathe and repeat on the left side. Option: With flexible wrists

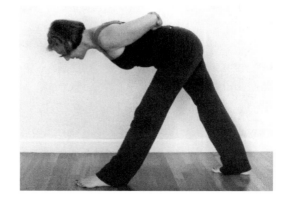

and shoulders you can bring the hands into clasped fists and straighten the arms. Extending the arms toward the ground behind you as you stand, raise them toward the ceiling as you fold. Additionally, with very open shoulders and flexible wrists, you may put hands in reverse prayer, palm against palm, fingertips to ceiling. Pulling elbows back toward each other and shoulder blades together, opening the heart, come into the pose. You may also bring the arms forward, putting the hands on the shins, ankles, or the ground in another variation of this hamstring-opening pose.

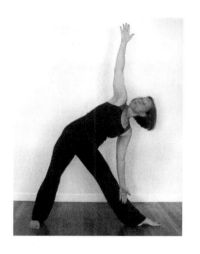

Triangle pose (*utthita trikonasana*). From *tadasana*, step the right foot back, heel farther toward the back of the mat than the toes; turn the body so that the hip bones face the long right side of the mat. Raise the arms parallel to the floor; left arms toward the front of the mat, right arm to the back, shoulders and shoulder blades lowering down the back. Take the right hip back toward the right leg and reach the left arm to the front of the mat, keeping the arms parallel to the floor until you have reached your farthest point. Then tip toward the floor, bringing the left hand to the inside of the left knee, calf, or ankle, or to the floor. Breathe as you rotate your chest up and tuck your right hip under. Press firmly into the feet to free the breath. Stay for a few breaths, come up, bringing hands to waist, and return the right foot to the left at the top of the mat. Breathe here a few times and experience your exertion. Repeat on the left side.

Extreme side angle pose (*utthita parsvakonasana*). From *tadasana*, step the right foot back, heel farther toward the back of the mat than the toes, and turn the body so that the hip bones face the long right side of the mat. Bringing the arms up parallel to the floor, bend the left knee until it comes over the left ankle. Using your core, bend the left elbow and place the left forearm at the elbow on the left knee. (If you are used to this pose you may reach the left hand to the floor either on the outside or the inside of the left foot. Use a block if the left arm does not reach the floor comfortably.) Reach the right arm up toward the ceiling and then over the right ear, stretching it toward the front of the mat. Stack the shoulders one above the other. Let your gaze be straight forward or, if the neck is flexible, gaze toward your right armpit. Keep the heart open and breathe smoothly and deeply a few rounds. Pushing into the feet, come up out of the extension, bring

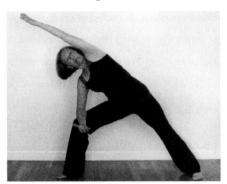

the arms down, and return the right foot to the front of the mat, coming into *tadasana*. Stand and absorb the sensations from the pose for a few breaths. Repeat on the left side.

Warrior pose I (*virahabdrasana* I). From standing mountain, *tadasana*, step the right foot back, right foot at a forty-five- to sixty-degree angle (toes pointing more forward than sideways), hip bones and chest facing forward. Extend the feet strongly into the mat, bend the left knee over the left ankle as you raise the arms forward, then reach overhead with palms parallel to each other. Moving the lower ribs away from the hip bones, letting the chest rise skyward, shoulder blades moving into and down the back, keep energy rising through the hands into the air. Keep the lower back moving away from the shoulders for a long, extended spine. If the neck is supple and loose the gaze can be focused toward the thumbs, or the gaze can remain in a forward-facing direction. If the shoulders become loose and open, the hands can move to palms-touching position. Remain in this pose for three to five breaths.

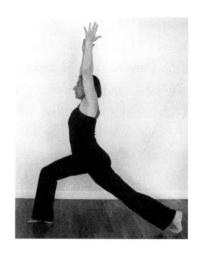

Return the arms to the sides, straighten the front knee, and draw the right leg forward to the front of the mat, resuming standing mountain pose (*tadasana*). Breathe here, then repeat on the other side.

Warrior pose II (*virahabdrasana* II). From standing mountain, *tadasana*, step the right foot back, right heel farther toward the back of the mat than the toes, and turn the body so that the hip bones face the long (right) side of the mat. Raise the arms parallel to the floor, shoulders and shoulder blades lowering down the back. Bend the left knee over the left ankle. Continue the descending energy by moving the lower back and sacrum away from the shoulders. From the waist, keep the energy moving down to the feet and up through the crown of the head.

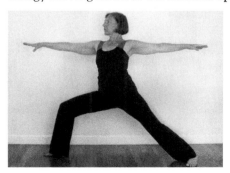

Breathe in steadiness. Hold for several breaths then drop the arms to the sides, straighten the left knee, and return the right leg to the front of the mat. Breathe and repeat on the left side.

Warrior III (*virahabdrasana* III). Move into warrior I from standing mountain (*tadasana*). From warrior I pose, right leg back, bring the arms forward at the same time you are transferring your weight to the left leg. Drag the toe of the right foot forward as you tip over the top of the supporting left leg. When ready, lift the right leg up parallel to the mat, lengthening and straightening the standing leg. Using the strength of the core muscles, extend the arms away from you as you press through the right heel, extending the right leg behind you with vigor. Face either the ground or directly in front of you, finding that focus point that will allow the gaze and the pose to be steady. Breathe several rounds, then descend the way you ascended, by softening the knee of the standing leg and bringing the arms overhead as the right leg returns to the mat and moves back, returning you to warrior I pose. Close the pose in the usual way, dropping the arms and bringing the back leg to the front of the mat into standing mountain (*tadasana*). Breathe here a few times before moving to the pose on the other side.

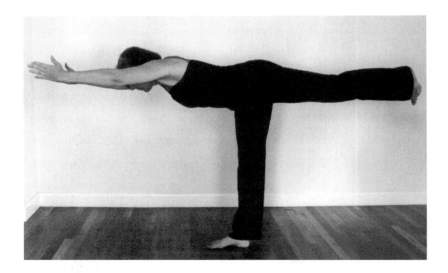

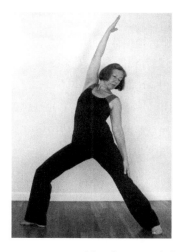

Reverse warrior II (*utthita virahabdrasana* II). Beginning in standing mountain (*tadasana*), move into warrior II pose. From the warrior II pose with right leg back, drop the right arm back to palm down on the right thigh. Raise the left arm skyward. Turning the head to face the right leg, bring the gaze to the right ankle. Feel the stretch along the left side of the body as you reach the left arm over and back toward the back of the mat. Ground through both feet. Breathe here three to five rounds. Return to warrior II pose, then drop the arms back to the sides, bringing the back foot forward, and come into standing mountain (*tadasana*). Repeat on the left side after a few breaths.

Chair pose (*utkatansana*). From standing mountain (*tadasana*), bring the feet a few inches apart, ensuring the toes are pointed forward. Raise the arms overhead and sit back into chair pose. Move the thumbs behind you, stretching and opening the shoulders. Keeping the legs parallel to each other, reach forward with the arms and reach back with the hips; hold for five to ten breaths. Return to standing mountain pose (*tadasana*). Repeat two more times.

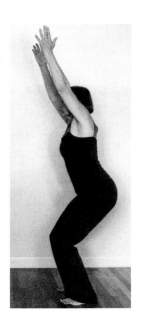

Downward-facing dog pose (*adho mukha svanasana*). From quadruped position, tuck the toes and, pushing into the arms, lengthen the spine and hips up to the sky. Let the head hang relaxed and loose, facing your thighs. Pushing strongly into the hand, into the "L" created by your thumb and forefinger, move the heel toward the floor, the shoulders moving to the hips, away from the ears, the hips continuing to move up toward the sky. If the hamstrings are tight, allow the knees

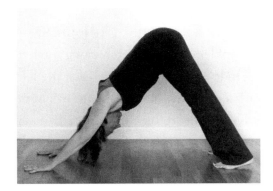

to remain soft. Breathe deeply three to five full breath cycles and enjoy the stretch. Return to hands and knees pose. Rest in child's pose if you wish. Repeat several times.

Standing forward fold pose (*uttanasana*). From *tadasana*, with hands on hips, fold from the hip crease and bend forward. Bring the hands to your thighs, your shins, a block on the mat, or the ground. Tip the hips forward and lengthen the back, breathing into the pose for half a minute or more. To come out, engage the core muscles of the torso, returning the hands to the hips; push into the heels, tuck the tail, and come straight up. Take a few breaths here and repeat.

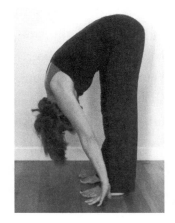

Standing back bend (*anuvittasana*), variation.
Starting in standing mountain pose (*tadasana*), bring the hands to the chest in prayer position (*anjali mudra*). Raise the arms above the head, shoulder width apart. Tightening the glutes, bring the hips slightly forward as you lengthen your spine and arch your back. Keep the ears in line with the biceps, bringing the gaze upward. Breathe. Using an inhale to return to upward salute with arms above head, exhale, bringing

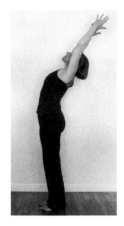

the hands back in front of the heart. Drop the hands back to the sides in standing mountain (*tadasana*). Breathe here a few times.

Tree pose (*vrikshasana*). From standing mountain (*tadasana*), bring the hands to the hips. Find a spot to focus on, a spot that does not move. This steady focal point will assist you in holding your balance. Transfer the weight to the left foot, bringing the right knee up

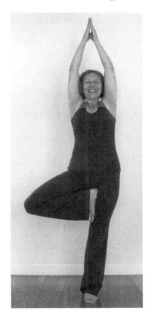

parallel to the ground; rotate the leg to the right and bring sole of the right foot to the inner thigh, shin, or ankle (avoid putting the sole on the knee; a misstep during balancing could cause damage to the supporting knee). Bring the hands in front of the heart in prayer position and then raise them above the head with palms either together or shoulder distance apart. Stay here for five to ten full breaths. Come out of the pose by bringing the hands in front of the heart, then return the right foot to the ground. Stand in *tadasana* for a few breaths, then repeat on the left side.

Cobra (bhujangasana), variation. From front-lying position, place the hands, fingers forward, next to the upper ribs, fingertips just below the shoulders. Point the elbows to the ceiling, drawing them together behind the back. Using the muscles of the back, raise the chest off the floor. Gaze forward and hold for a few breaths. Only look up if your neck is comfortable. If you have a flexible back, you may use the strength of the arms to increase the arc. If you do not have as flexible a back, your pose may result in your chest coming only a few inches off the mat. This is your pose. Feel the breath move the torso up and down. Return to face-down pose, one cheek on the mat, after five to ten breaths and repeat a few times, alternating which cheek you return to the mat after each round.

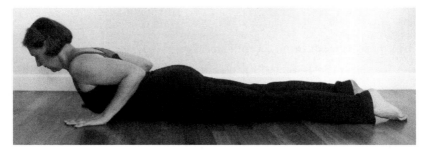

Staff or seated mountain pose (dandasana). Come into straight-legged sitting position, walking the legs forward on the mat so that you are on your sit bones. Flex the feet and move the backs of the knees toward the mat. Lengthen the spine from the mat through the back of the neck to the crown of the head. Bring the hands palms down, fingers forward, to the mat near the hips. Push out through the heels, push through the arms into the flexed hands, and lengthen the spine. Breathe and grow tall and long. Hold for three to five breaths. Release.

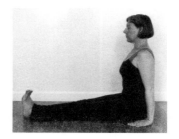

Upward-facing boat pose (*paripurna navasana*). From a seated position, bend the knees, putting the soles of the feet on the mat. Holding the backs of the thighs with the hands, straighten and

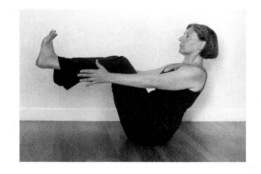

lengthen the back. Engage the abdominals and tip back to balance on the sit bones. Extend the lower legs, bringing the shins parallel to the floor. Reinvigorate the abdominals and extend the hands toward the ankles. If you like, you may extend through the heels, pushing out until the legs are straight. Breathe and hold for ten breaths. Any step along the way in this pose is a perfect modification. Find your way to the full pose with compassion and effort.

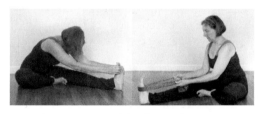

Single-legged, seated, forward fold (*janu sirsasana*). From a tall balanced staff or seated mountain (*dandasana*) position with the legs outstretched, bring the sole of the right foot to the inside of the left thigh. Raising the arms overhead, folding from the hips, elongate the upper body forward over the extended left leg. Drop the hands to the knee, then shin, then ankle, or ring them around the sole of the extended left foot. Use a strap or belt around the sole of the left foot to keep the spine straight before surrendering into the fold. Breathe and hold for ten cycles. Return to seated position and extend the right leg into seated mountain. Breathe and then move into the stretch on the left side. Return to seated mountain and breathe to integrate the stretch. Repeat on the other side.

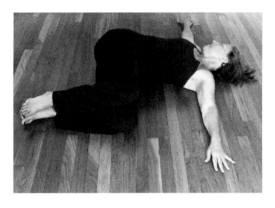

Simple twist (*jathara parivartasana*). From back-lying position, extend the arms directly out from the shoulders into a "T" position. Draw the knees to the chest then drop them over to the right side toward the right elbow. If comfortable, you may turn the head to the left. Breathe into the back, body, and belly. Stay here for ten breaths. Engage the abdominals, bringing the knees back to the chest and lowering them to the left. Return to deep breaths for an equal length of time. (Variation: Extend the legs once the twist is completed to each side, bending them again before changing sides.) Return to back-lying pose. After the second side, extend the legs one at a time and take a few breaths to experience the body sensations.

Corpse pose (*savasana*). Lying on the back, with knees bent, feet flat on the floor, bring the arms along the sides, resting the palms up next to the hips. Pushing into the hips and the upper edge of the shoulders, lift the midback slightly and draw the shoulder blades just a little closer to each other, opening the chest. Extend the legs

along the mat one at a time, allowing them to separate about mat distance apart. Fully relax the feet, allowing them to tip out. Close the eyes and soften behind the eyelids. Soften all the muscles of the head, face,

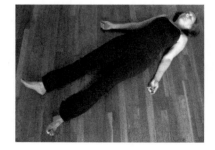

neck, throat, and chest; let go completely. Remain like this for five to twenty minutes. Come out slowly by first stretching, then bringing knees to chest, and roll onto the right side. Allow the strength of the arms to help you return to any comfortable seated position. Bring the hands in front of the heart and recall your intention. Namaste.

APPENDIX IV

The Principles of the Twelve Steps

All twelve-step programs follow the same Twelve Steps first developed by Bill Wilson and Dr. Robert Smith, a pair of alcoholics considered the founders of Alcoholics Anonymous, the "great-grandaddy" program of twelve-step recovery. Though the wording may differ slightly from fellowship to fellowship, the principles are exactly the same. A generic version of the steps and principles common to virtually all twelve-step programs of recovery is provided below.

STEP ONE: Requires one to admit one's powerlessness— over substances, behaviors, other people, events, etc., as well as make an acknowledgment that one's life has become unmanageable. Principles: acceptance and surrender.

STEP TWO: Involves the realization that a power greater than oneself can restore one to mental, physical, and spiritual health. Principles: faith and hope.

STEP THREE: Calls for a decision to turn one's life and will over to the care of a Higher Power. Principles: trust and commitment.

STEP FOUR: Demands a thorough review and assessment of past wrongs committed by the person taking the step. Principles: honesty and courage.

STEP FIVE: Requires an admission of those wrongs, first by acknowledgment to oneself, then to the Higher Power, and finally, to another person. Principles: trust and commitment.

STEP SIX: Necessitates making a conscious choice to have the character defects revealed in Steps Four and Five removed by one's Higher Power. Principle: willingness.

STEP SEVEN: Requires that one make a sincere request to have the character flaws removed by one's Higher Power. Principle: faith.

STEP EIGHT: Involves making a list of all those one has wronged and accepting the need to make those wrongs right. Principle: responsibility.

STEP NINE: Requires that amends must be made to all those one has harmed, except when to make amends would cause further harm to the injured party or to others. Principles: restitution and reparation, whether directly or indirectly; also responsibility and acceptance of consequences.

STEP TEN: Suggests a daily examination of conscience in order to discover any ongoing wrongdoings or character flaws. Principles: commitment, discipline.

STEP ELEVEN: Calls for ongoing prayer and meditation with the purpose of maintaining and improving a "god-consciousness" (or building spirituality) in the life of the recovering person. Principle: spiritual growth.

STEP TWELVE: Performance of the steps helps to lead one to a "spiritual awakening," as a result of which the now-recovering person understands that he or she must help others who suffer from the same disease/disorder. Principle: repayment, altruism.

If you would like to learn more about how these steps are adapted to specific programs of recovery, you may find twelve-step recovery groups in most phone books or online, listed alphabetically by the name of the substance/behavior they primarily address, e.g., Narcotics Anonymous, Alcoholics Anonymous, or Gamblers Anonymous. These groups also maintain websites and hotlines. Typically, houses of worship, social service agencies, and treatment centers can also provide information. For many who suffer with addiction, the Twelve Steps have proven to be the key to a happy, healthy, and fulfilling life.